Contents

Health and behaviour: Selected perspectives

Edited by

David Hamburg

Carnegie Corporation of New York,
437 Madison Avenue, New York NY 10022

Norman Sartorius

Division of Mental Health, World Health Organization,
CH-1211, Geneva 27, Switzerland

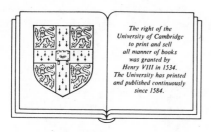

The right of the
University of Cambridge
to print and sell
all manner of books
was granted by
Henry VIII in 1534.
The University has printed
and published continuously
since 1584.

Published on behalf of the World Health

Organization by

CAMBRIDGE UNIVERSITY PRESS

Cambridge

New York   Port Chester   Melbourne   Sydney

Published by the Press Syndicate of the University of Cambridge
The Pitt Building, Trumpington Street, Cambridge CB2 1RP
40 West 20th Street, New York, NY 10011, USA
10 Stamford Road, Oakleigh, Melbourne 3166, Australia

© Cambridge University Press 1989

First published 1989

Printed in Great Britain at the University Press, Cambridge

British Library CIP data available

Library of Congress cataloguing in publication data

Health and behaviour.

Includes index.
1. Medicine and psychology. 2. Social medicine.
I. Hamburg, David A., 1925–   . II. Sartorius, N.
[DNLM: 1. Attitude to Health. 2. Behaviour—psychology.
3. Mental Disorders—psychology. 4. Psychology, Social.
5. Psychophysiologic Disorders. W 85 H434]
R726.5.H432 1989 610'.19 88–29711
ISBN 0 521 36352 7

CUP 1014 /32.50 · 4.91

UP

List of contributors

Chapters 1 and 6

Dr Heinz Häfner, Zentralinstitut für Seelische Gesundheit, 68 Mannheim J5, FRG

Dr Rainer Welz, Department of Medical Sociology, University of Göttingen, Humboldt-Allee 3, Göttingen, FRG

Chapter 2

Dr M. Abdussalam, c/o World Health Organization, CH-1211, Geneva 27, Switzerland

Professor C. Foster, Department of Anthropology, University of California, Berkeley, California, USA

Dr F. Käferstein, Division of Environmental Health, World Health Organization, CH-1211, Geneva 27, Switzerland

Chapter 3

Dr T. Wachs, Department of Psychological Sciences, Purdue University, West Lafayette, Indiana 47907, USA

Chapter 4

Professor P. Graham, Institute for Child Health, Hospital for Sick Children, Great Ormond Street, London, WC1, UK

Chapter 5

Professor B. A. Hamburg, Department of Psychiatry and Pediatrics, Mount Sinai School of Medicine, 1 Gustav L. Levy Place, New York, NY 10029, USA

Chapter 7
Professor D. Goldberg, Department of Psychiatry, University of Manchester, Manchester, UK

Chapter 8
Professor D. Banerji, Centre of Social Medicine and Community Health, Jawaharlal Nehru University, New Delhi 11067, India

Chapter 9
Dr Patricia L. Rosenfield, Carnegie Corporation of New York, 437 Madison Avenue, New York, NY 10022, USA

Chapter 10
Professor D. Hamburg, Carnegie Corporation of New York, 437 Madison Avenue, New York, NY 10022, USA
Professor N. Sartorius, Division of Mental Health, World Health Organization, CH-1211, Geneva 27, Switzerland

Preface

Human behaviour is a key to health, and changes in behaviour have a profound influence on patterns of morbidity, and mortality from disease.

This fact is not a new discovery. From the earliest days of human history, behaviour has been the focus of most of the action aiming to prevent and treat illness. Dietary and hygienic prescriptions are embedded in most religions and rituals of mourning are undertaken by the bereaved to help them overcome stress. Societal relations are regulated to strengthen supportive social networks. In the past, links between behavioural change and the course of disease were frequently not well understood, and behavioural action was recommended because of the correlations observed − recommended nevertheless with force and insistence.

The twentieth century brought with it clear evidence of causal links between specific forms of behaviour − including attitudes, action and comprehension − and improvement or deterioration of health states. An impressive amount of literature has been produced over the past decades in this area, and both the public and the scientific community have become acutely aware of the need to influence behaviour if progress is to be made in promoting health, preventing disease, or decreasing suffering of those in whom it has appeared. Insistence that appropriate action be taken has not only stemmed from scientists; government leaders have also addressed the question. The World Health Assembly, bringing together chief health executives from 160 member states, for example, has devoted much of its time to the discussion of this matter. The results were resolutions of the Assembly requesting action in member states and internationally.

The World Health Organization's programme on biobehavioural sciences and mental health has been created to initiate international action and support national efforts. Among its various activities, raising awareness of the links between behaviour and health has a key role. This book is a part of that effort. It aims to draw attention to aspects of the relationships between behaviour and health which have received insufficient attention in recent years. Selection of these perspectives has been made easier by several recent publications providing coverage of a number of important issues (e.g. Hamburg *et al.*, 1982).

The programme on biobehavioural sciences and mental health is an initiative which could not survive without contributions from many research centres and individuals across the world. Funds for the programme have been obtained from the budget of WHO, and from contributions by several governments and foundations, notably from the Carnegie Corporation of New York. It is our pleasant duty to thank all of them and to express the hope that they will continue participating in the work of the Organization on this topic, joined by many others who believe in the possibility of improving health through behavioural interventions stemming from a conscious and willing participation of people in the improvement of their health.

David Hamburg
Norman Sartorius

Acknowledgements

The editors acknowledge with gratitude the contributions made by Mrs Betty Appelbaum who has copy-edited the manuscript so conscientiously and with so much patience, Professor Philip Graham who gave us many valuable comments, Dr Elena Nightingale, for clarifying important substantive issues, and Mrs Anne Yamada who took care of the many administrative chores connected with this work, checked the proofs, collated the corrections of the various authors and made most useful suggestions about the book as a whole.

Abbreviations

AIDS Acquired Immune Deficiency Syndrome
DIS Diagnostic Interview Schedule
DSM-III Diagnostic and statistical manual of mental disorders, third edition
FELDA Federal Land Development Authority
ICD-9 *International classification of diseases*, ninth edition
NIMH National Institute of Mental Health of the USA
PEEM Panel of Experts on Environmental Management for Vector Control
PEM Protein-energy malnutrition
PHCs Primary Health Centres
PHS Public Health Services
PSE Present State Examination
RDC Research Diagnostic Criteria
RMPs Registered Medical Practitioners
SEARO South-East Asia Regional Office, WHO
SISS Suicide Intention and Seriousness Scale

1

Social and behavioural determinants of mental disorders

Heinz Häfner and Rainer Welz

The broad scope and the seriousness of the burden of illness directly associated with behaviour have been recognized as a major problem of public health and health policy. Between behaviour and related illness there is a great diversity of associations, which can be differentiated according to three aspects: health-relevant behaviour, which, in the form of risk behaviour, influences the probability of falling physically ill (e.g overt patterns of health-damaging behaviour such as smoking, faulty nutrition, and insufficient sanitary practices); identification of illness with deviant behaviour; and, finally, behavioural patterns or disabilities that result from illness and thus constitute a burden in themselves.

A major category in the behaviour-relevant burden of illness is overt mental illness. There are about 100 million people in the world who suffer from depressive disorders, and 40 million from other psychotic disorders. Another sizeable category in the burden of behaviour-related illness includes minor mental disorders, substance abuse, and drinking problems.

In many cases, chronic physical ill health and mental disorder interact. Chronic physical illnesses and disabilities frequently have an impact on patients' mental health, thus increasing the utilization of, and burden upon, the primary groups of the social network. When combined with physical illness, mental disorder may entail neglect of necessary dietary regimes or the intake of prescribed medicines and thus lead to a further deterioration in the patient's health. Other examples of how behavioural patterns may increase the risk of mental and physical illness are substance abuse and chronic alcohol abuse.

For the purpose of prevention and treatment of mental disorders and thus prevention and reduction of the related burden, it is essential to know the factors that influence their genesis, course, and outcome. Not only genetic factors and

Professor Dr Dr Häfner is Head of the Zentralinstitut für Seelische Gesundheit, PO Box 122120, D-6800 Mannheim FRG. Dr Welz, who was formerly with the same institute, is now with the Department of Medical Psychology, University of Göttingen, Humboldt-Allee, 3 Göttingen, FRG.

gical and biochemical processes but also psychological and social factors
be taken into account.

regard to ecological factors, a distinction needs to be made between those
reflected in incidence rates and influence the risk of mental illness in a great
many people, on the one hand, and those that, on the other hand, operate only at
the level of smaller social groups and influence the risk in a small number of people.
Examples of highly general factors, ones influencing the risk of falling ill in large
collectives, are culture-related behaviour patterns, such as alcohol consumption,
and risk factors pertaining to socio-economic status. Social groups, such as family,
peer group, or the social network of friends and acquaintances in a residential area,
are examples of less general factors that seem to influence the individual risk of
mental illness.

In what follows, while focusing on the psychosocial factors influencing the risk,
onset, course, and outcome of mental disorders, we shall not exclude the possible
influence of biological factors.

Even in such clear-cut cases of environment-related mental disorder as
alcoholism and chronic alcohol abuse, the variation in incidence rates across
societies is, at least to some extent, attributable to genetic factors, as shown, for
example, by the studies conducted by Reed & co-workers (1) on the mechanisms
governing the metabolism of alcohol in Europeans and Asians.

The first stage in the metabolism of alcohol in the organism is the oxidation to
acetaldehyde and acetate under the influence of the enzyme alcohol dehydrogenase
(ADH), which acts mainly in the liver. An iso-enzyme of ADH – first described by
Wartburg, Papenburg & Aebi (2) – which is found in 5% of the European
population (3), effects a rapid increase in acetaldehyde in the plasma because of
its higher activity. The enzymatic breakdown of acetaldehyde by aldehyde
dehydrogenase is part of the second stage (4). Even a deficit of this enzyme, which
seems to be the case in the majority of Japanese (5) and Chinese, will cause a rise
in the plasma level of acetaldehyde, which can cause unpleasant symptoms in
drinkers of alcohol. The most common of these symptoms are flushing, palpitations,
and increased blood pressure. Propping (6) has recently criticized the culture-
related explanations of the less common occurrence of alcoholism in Asiatic
countries than in Europe by stating that, because of the genetic peculiarities of the

metabolism of alcohol, members of the Mongoloid races may well be better
protected against excessive drinking.

The opposite is the case in physical dependence on heroin. In spite of being
based on biochemical and physiological processes in the organism, the risk of
persistent use can be decisively influenced by psychosocial factors. This is
suggested by an investigation conducted by Robins (7, 8) on Americans who had
fought in the Vietnam War; only 9% of the soldiers who had taken heroin
regularly and developed dependence continued to take the drug after returning to

the United States. In this group, subjects who had grown up in socially deprived residential areas and disrupted families were overrepresented. Their parents had had excessive drinking habits, and the men themselves had displayed deviant behaviour at an early age.

These two examples illustrate the interaction between biological and psychosocial factors, operant even in behavioural disorders that have so far been attributed almost exclusively to either psychosocial or biological factors.

Though most of the research on the concurrence of biological, social, and psychological factors has been done in developed countries, the data on appearance, course, rehabilitation, and prevention of behaviour-related illnesses are independent of cultural variables. They are valid for developing countries as well, even though these countries often differ from one another and from developed countries with respect to their cultural and social context and their health care systems.

The incidence of mental disorders
Mental disorders in general practice

Given the great diversity of mental disorders and minor psychological disturbances and their varying frequences, it is difficult to obtain exact information on their incidence, distribution, and the related burden they represent. To achieve ideal results in investigating these questions, direct studies on unselected populations should be carried out. Field studies and investigations of representative samples are, however, associated with high costs and are expedient only if the size of the group under study corresponds to the expected frequency of the features of interest.

A good way of obtaining data on and indicators of mental morbidity is to investigate the clientele of general practitioners (GPs). The prerequisite for such studies is the participation of all the GPs providing care for a defined population or a sample of the GPs serving an area. The clientele of GPs is fairly representative in areas where free treatment is provided for the entire population and where a dense network of primary physicians is available. According to Shepherd & co-workers (9), approximately 95% of the total population in Great Britain is registered with GPs, and about 60% of those registered consult their family doctors at least once a year. In their study, Shepherd and colleagues arrived at a first-consultation rate of 139.4/1000 adult population for 46 general practices in London.

In the Federal Republic of Germany, two general-practice studies have been conducted. One was carried out by Dilling, Weyerer & Enders (10) in Upper Bavaria, and the second, by Zintl-Wiegand & Cooper (11) in Mannheim, on the basis of the clientele of 18 and 13 general practices, respectively. A sample of patients who had come to consult their family doctors were, in addition to being treated by the GPs, examined by a research psychiatrist. The 14-day prevalence rate of patients with a psychiatric diagnosis was 32% for Upper Bavaria and 35.5% for Mannheim. Since mentally ill persons, particularly patients with neurotic symptoms, generally consult physicians more often than mentally healthy persons do (*12, 13*), these figures represent an overestimate of the proportion of mentally ill.

In the overwhelming majority of the patients diagnosed as suffering from a mental disorder or disturbance, both physical and mental symptoms are present. This is due either to the simultaneous presence of more than one disease or to illnesses producing both physical and the mental symptoms, such as drug dependence leading to liver damage, or anxiety neurosis in conjunction with paroxysmal tachycardia. Only 7% of the patients diagnosed as mentally disordered received no additional somatic diagnosis from the GPs in the study conducted by Dilling & colleagues (*10*).

When generalizing on the basis of general-practice studies, it must be taken into account that the data on rare and severe illnesses may not be representative, because the probability of such cases occurring in the group under study is too low and the persons affected turn directly to hospitals and other specialist services. Therefore, general-practice studies allow generalizations mainly on frequently occurring minor mental disorders, such as milder depressions, neurotic and reactive syndromes, and milder brain syndromes in old age.

Case-register studies

In contrast to general-practice studies, case-register studies focus on severe mental disorders.

Case registers are of preeminent importance, considering the fact that of the psychiatric services operating in a particular area, as many as possible (in an ideal case, all) contribute to the collection of information on treated cases. According to Wing & Fryers (*14*), case registers have the following three characteristics:

1. They represent documentation systems collecting, in a central register, the information on individuals provided by various health services, such as hospitals, outpatient services, or private psychiatrists.
2. They cover populations ranging from 100 000 to 1 million in geographically defined regions.
3. They are cumulative over several years.

The simplest purpose for which psychiatric case registers can be used is to provide answers to questions such as, which population segments currently utilize psychiatric services, and for what illnesses or to what extent do the utilization patterns suggest certain developments. The psychiatric case registers so far evaluated (*15–18*) have shown annual frequency rates of contacts with mental health services to be remarkably constant, ranging from 1.5% to 3.6% of the populations at risk. Case registers also enable continuous investigation and documentation of changes in the utilization of psychiatric services. Hence, they can be employed in the planning and evaluation of new mental health services and programmes.

It was with the help of a psychiatric case register that Häfner & Klug (*19*) investigated changes in the utilization of psychiatric services in connection with the transition from a hospital-centred to an integrated, community-based service structure. They were able to show that the work load of all the services of the community mental health system increased. The increase was most distinct in the outpatient sector and in the emergency and crisis intervention services. In these areas the more extensive availability of care covered needs previously unmet. The distribution by diagnoses revealed that help requested and provided for minor mental disorders – depressive states – psychotic and non-psychotic, and alcohol-related disorders increased most, whereas care of patients with dementia or mentally retarded patients with psychiatric diagnoses did not show any clear increase.

Field and community studies

A great advantage of case registers is the comprehensive and continuous registration of all contacts with all mental health services by a defined population and a somewhat narrower scope of case definitions, based on diagnoses given by psychiatrists from a limited number of cooperating mental health facilities in a defined catchment area. But studies conducted at the level of psychiatric services are marred by the fact that they do not provide any information from general practitioners and other non-psychiatric health services or on the amount of untreated mental morbidity in the general population. The proportion of untreated cases varies with the diagnosis: it is low for schizophrenia and considerably higher for minor mental disorders.

In developing countries lacking comprehensive health care systems, assessment of mental morbidity on the basis of utilization data is not feasible; in these countries field and community studies are the only means of obtaining information on untreated cases. The methods employed differ greatly, including interviews of so-called key informants, such as teachers or community nurses, on the one hand, and medical or psychiatric examinations with or without screening, on the other.

The selected field studies (see Table 1) differ considerably in terms of their results achieved in different countries and areas. The rates ascertained for mental disorder in the general population range from 4 % in Vaucluse (France) (*20*) to 55 % in the Stirling County study (Canada) (*21*). The reasons for the variation are multifarious, including differences in case definition, in the size and repre-sentativeness of the samples, and in the prevalence periods chosen. Higher rates

Table 1. *Psychiatric morbidity among general population as related to case definition and case identification (per 100 000)*

Case identification: medical examination, in part supplemented by interviews of key persons and analysis of medical records		Questionnaires and structured interviews							Semi-standardized instruments	
		Health opinion survey		Mental health scale		Other instruments of interview				
Roth & Luton (24)	12.3	Leighton et al. (21)	55.0	Srole et al. (40)	23.4	Cole et al. (48)	30.0		Dohrenwend (58)	21.79
Bremer (25)	20.8	Edgerton et al. (36)	24.0	Phillips (41)	27.5	Brunetti (49)	39.7		Weissman et al. (59)	17.8
Fremming (26)	11.9	Schwab (34)	30.4	Hease & Meile (42)	44.0	Taylor & Chave (50)	33.0		Wing et al. (60)	19.0
Essen-Möller (27)	8.1	Shore (38)	54.0	Meile & Hease (43)	32.3	Hare & Shaw (51)	24.13		Finlay-Jones & Burvill (61)	16.0
Trussell (28)	18.0	Schwab et al. (39)	29.0	Phillips & Segal et al. (44)	28.4	Piotrowski et al. (52)	10.5			
Pasamanick et al. (29)	12.83			Summers et al. (45)	16.6		8.3		Shiraer & Armstrong (62)	13.0
Llewellyn-Thomas (30)	55.8			Gaitz & Scott (46)	33.6	Giel & Le Nobel (53)	15.0		Henderson (63)	27.4
				Yancey et al. (47)	31.8	Schwab & Warheit (54)	31.1		Leaf et al. (64)	17.4
Primrose (31)	13.17					Bjarnar et al. (55)	20.5			
Helgason (32)	28.6					Väisänen (56)	28.2			
Hagnell (33)	16.0					Schepank (57)	27.1			
Brunetti (20)	4.11									
	6.11									
Andersen (34)	13.85									
	18.95									
Fugelli (35)	29.11									
Median	13.17		30.4		28.4		27.1			17.8

Based on Dohrenwend *et al.* (23), and supplemented by the authors.

are obtained if a broad case definition is applied, if the surveys are conducted on risk groups, and, if earlier cases inactive at the time of study are included than if the case definition is narrow, the sample is representative, and inactive cases are excluded. For a review, see Dohrenwend & Dohrenwend (22) and Dohrenwend & associates (23).

As mentioned above, the findings depend on the methods employed in case identification and case definition. In the studies included in Table 1, we can distinguish a number of methods of case identification: personal medical examination, in part supplemented by interviews of key informants and an analysis of case notes; structured interviews; and semi- or completely standardized interviews, such as the Present State Examination (PSE), Research Diagnostic Criteria (RDC), or the NIMH Diagnostic Interview Schedule (DIS).

If the prevalence rates ascertained in the studies are grouped together according to the method used in case definition and the median is calculated, the median increases as we move from a narrow to a broad case definition. For cases identified by means of a medical examination, the median is 13.17%; for clinical interviews, 17.6%; and for other studies in which questionnaires were used, the figure ranges between 27.1% and 30.4%.

Irrespective of case definition and the heterogeneity of the samples, the overall median for the studies is 18.95%. The studies conducted by Wing & co-workers (60) and Weissman, Myers & Harding (59) show that this figure gives a fairly realistic picture of the actual occurrence of mental disorder in the general population. Wing & colleagues, in London, were the first to conduct field studies in which a semistandardized diagnostic instrument, validated on clinical populations and samples drawn from the general population, was used for case identification. By means of this instrument (the PSE), they found that the proportion of mentally disturbed persons was 19%. Weissman & associates, using the RDC, found that 17.6% of the subjects interviewed suffered from a mental disorder. In a more recent study, which they conducted together with Leaf & co-workers (64) and in which they used the NIMH Diagnostic Interview Schedule in diagnosing on the basis of DSM-III (65) criteria, they arrived at an approximately equally high proportion of mental disorders (17.4%) in the adult population. Age constitutes one of the most important variables of the risk of mental illness. Since a high proportion of the elderly is placed in homes or hospitals, the results presented in Table 1 are valid only for the adult population up to the age of 65.

Direct investigations of elderly populations

Epidemiological cross-sectional studies on elderly people living in private households, in homes for the elderly, or in hospitals, or on elderly populations at large, as independent studies or in connection with large-scale epidemiological surveys, have been conducted in many countries (for a review, see Häfner,

Table 2. Prevalence of mental disorder in the population aged over 65: estimates from field studies (%)

Authors	Survey area	Number of persons	Organic psychoses	Milder organic syndromes	Functional psychoses	Neuroses and personality disorders	Total[a]
Sheldon (68)	Wolverhampton, UK (urban)	369	3.9	11.7	—	12.6	28.2
Primrose (31)	N. Scotland (rural)	222	4.5	—	1.4	12.6	—
Nielsen (70)	Samsø Island (rural)	978	3.1	15.4	3.7	6.8	29.0
Kay et al. (71)	Newcastle, UK (urban)	443	5.7	5.7	2.4	12.5	26.3
Parsons (72)	Swansea, UK (urban)	228	4.4	—	2.6	4.8	—
Dilling & Weyerer (73)	Upper Bavaria, FRG (semi-rural)	295	8.5	8.5	3.4	10.2	23.1
Cooper & Sosna (68)	Mannheim, FRG (urban)	519	6.0	5.4	2.2	10.8	24.4

[a] Totals given include only cases in the four broad categories listed. In the Samsø and Newcastle surveys, higher prevalence estimates, which include various borderline groups, are also given.
Source: Cooper (66).

Moschel, & Sartorius [*18*]). Although they have differed somewhat in case definitions and assessment methods, the overall results are of the same order of magnitude. In about one-fifth to one-fourth of those aged 65 and above, mental disorders or psychological disturbances were found to be present at the time of investigation (*66, 67*). A study conducted on a representative sample of 65 year-old Mannheim inhabitants (*68*) revealed great differences between the frequency of mental disorders among the over 65 year-olds in private households and those in homes for the elderly or in hospital care: the frequency rate of mental disorder was 24.4% for the total elderly population, 41.8% for those placed in homes, and 23.3% for those living in private households.

An analysis according to diagnostic categories, i.e the presence of certain illness groups, showed that mental disorders relating from brain diseases or disturbances in brain functioning occupy first place in quantitative terms, followed by neuroses and related conditions. In comparison, functional psychosis, such as manic-depressive states or schizophrenias, are of diminishing importance (see Table 2); but this does not apply to the large group of 'non-psychotic' depressive disorders, subsumed under 'neuroses and personality disorders' in Table 2. This is true for all elderly populations on which methodologically high-standard, and thus informative, epidemiological studies have been conducted.

The most important disorders in old age, in quantitative and health policy terms, are the large group of depressive disorders and dementia, which, through a gradual loss of memory and intellectual functioning leads to mental disability and, finally, to need for care and nursing. A considerable proportion of the loss of intellectual powers diagnosed as organic psychosyndromes in early old age later results in dementia. Depressive disorders also constitute a risk factor for various physical illnesses and suicide.

The frequency of mental disorders increases steeply with age. Beyond the age of 85 it reaches very high rates. In organic psychosyndromes the rise is solely accounted for by dementia: the frequency of dementia is estimated at 20%–30% for the over 85 year-olds, compared with 2%–3% for the 65–69 year-olds (*74*). Studies conducted in Denmark (*70*), the Federal Republic of Germany (*69*), Great Britain (*75*), Japan (*76*), and the United States (*77*) indicate that the steep increase in the frequency of dementia in advanced age occurs in all the cultures studied. The frequency of functional mental disorders, particularly depressive illness, declines slightly in advanced age. This might be due to, among other factors, depressive disorders becoming erased by progressive dementia, or to a decrease in the proportion of the elderly with depressive disorders as a result of selective mortality. Depressive disorders are often associated with severe coronary heart disease and constitute a predictor of reduced life expectancy (*78*).

Chronic physical and mental illness

The interaction between chronic physical and mental illness has not yet been studied sufficiently, but there is reason to believe it to be closer than expected. One example is the relation between alcohol abuse and the development of alcohol delirium, cirrhosis of the liver, polyneuropathy, or alcohol-related brain atrophy. Investigations of patients in general practices (79) and the results of field studies (80) have shown that mentally ill persons exhibit more physical symptoms than corresponding control groups of mentally healthy individuals.

A field study carried out by Cooper & co-workers (81, 82) among persons over 65 in Mannheim revealed a high frequency of physical illness among the mentally ill compared with age-matched mentally healthy people. The ratio of the frequency of disturbances of vision and hearing and of impairment in mobility ranged between 2 to 1 and 3 to 1 between mentally ill and mentally healthy persons. The trend was more pronounced for organic syndromes than for functional disorders, but the difference did not reach the level of significance. The interrelation of mental illness and physical impairment and disability was observed in both males and females in all age groups over 65 irrespective of social class.

The proportion of patients admitted to mental hospitals while suffering from a physical impairment is between 27% and 46%, according to various studies (83–86). In some cases the proportion of mentally ill patients treated for physical impairment in general hospitals is even higher, ranging from 15% to 86% (87). The most common mental syndromes in physically ill people are depression, organic brain syndromes, and alcoholism (88–90). As for coronary heart disease, one of the most frequent physical illnesses and highly associated with mental morbidity, 64% of hospitalized cardiac patients were found to be depressed (91). In many cases such mental disorders persist and adversely influence rehabilitation.

The relation between mental and physical health in old age

The previously cited study that Cooper & Sosna (68) conducted among the Mannheim population over 65 years old and living in private accommodation revealed that 26% of the elderly suffered from moderate or severe impairment of mobility; 17%, from a comparable impairment of hearing; and 13%, from an impairment of vision. Overall, 9.6% of the subjects examined were assessed as suffering from a severe physical impairment, and 25.3%, from a moderate one; this means that 35% of the population over 65 and living in private accommodation were assessed as suffering from at least moderate physical impairment. Over two-thirds of the elderly rated as moderately or severely physically impaired, as opposed to one-tenth of the physically healthy, were diagnosed as mentally ill (see Table 3). With the increasing severity of physical impairment, the frequency of mental illness increased. The relationship is significant in both organic and functional physical disorders (92).

Table 3. *Physical impairment and mental illness* (%)

	Physical impairment		
	None (0)	Mild (1)	Moderate–severe (2–4)
Suffering from mental disorders	11.3	23.1	45.2
of which			
organic psycho-syndromes	1.5	14.7	20.2
functional mental disorders	9.8	8.4	25.0

Chi^2 (cases/non-cases) = 32.57, df = 2, $P < 0.001$.
Source: Based on Sosna (*92*).

Physical illness and disability constitute the main risk factors for mental health in old age. However, the direction and nature of this relation between physical and mental health are not uniform for all illnesses. In depressions, illness-related behaviour becomes important in terms of how the patient reacts to the mental strain caused by physical illness and the possible threat to his life. On the other hand, physical disabilities frequently exert an influence on the mental state and social activity of elderly people: defective hearing can substantially impede interpersonal communication, and impairment of mobility considerably restricts social contacts. Hence, great obstacles often arise to opportunities for enjoying life and experiencing esteem and support from contacts with other people. In many cases the ability to cope with such fundamental changes in life situation in old age is considerably reduced because of an absence of alternatives or the onset of regression processes. Thus, chronic physical illness or disabilities may lead to loss of coping abilities, to helplessness, hopelessness, and, finally, depression.

Psycho-organic syndromes due to cerebrovascular or senile atrophies of the brain can often be regarded as direct consequences of a basic physical disease. Optimal medical treatment or provision of the proper dietary regime in basic diseases such as old-age diabetes and hypertension represent important means of preventing subsequent mental disorders, above all, mental disorders resulting from deficits in brain functioning. The fundamental importance of this aspect is demonstrated by the results of a Swedish cohort study conducted by Svanborg & co-workers (*93*): physically healthy 70 year-olds showed no signs of intellectual decline. The above-mentioned physical illnesses constitute risk factors of decisive importance for the onset of dementia at higher ages.

The cited Swedish study (*93*) showed heavy smoking, a risk behaviour exerting an influence from earlier stages of life, to be associated with earlier onset of processes of intellectual decline in old age. As Svanborg suggests, the association is probably mediated through an elevated risk for cardiovascular and cerebrovascular diseases in heavy smokers. How complex these associations are, is illustrated by the fact that density of the skeleton, muscle strength, and gonadal function decline more rapidly in heavy smokers than in non-smokers in old age. The first two factors increase the risk for fractures, such as the greatly feared fracture of the neck of the femur, in elderly people. In contrast, a relative dominance of an elevated oestrogen activity in women and of an elevated androgenic activity in men in old age have been found to correlate with better intellectual functioning and better mental health (93).

The influence of culture on mental health
Cultural influences on services and their structure and utilization
Study of the influence of culture and related socio-economic factors on mental health is a complex task. It is advisable to investigate the influence of cultural factors not only on individual behaviour and the distribution of risk factors but also on attitudes toward mental illnesses, their definition, and treatment. Besides sociocultural differences, on which attitudes toward mental illnesses and their definition depend, the structure and capacity of mental health services largely determine who utilizes such services and, consequently, who is regarded as ill and in need of treatment.

As an example of the great differences in the structures of mental health systems, Figure 1 illustrates the range of psychiatric beds per 10 000 adult population in 34 countries. The figure also shows that there is a highly significant correlation between the bed ratio and per capita gross national product.

Although many developing countries have specialist psychiatric services, they frequently lack larger components of a modern community-based psychiatric service network, such as outpatient, complementary, and rehabilitation facilities and specialized services for particular risk groups (alcoholics, etc.). Developing countries often have neither enough trained personnel nor the financial resources to implement extended mental health care programmes, though the proportion of the population with mental disorders is the same as that in developed countries.

Sociocultural influences on the etiology of mental disorder
The incidence of mental disorders, particularly of behavioural disturbances such as attempted suicide, drug abuse, and alcoholism, is closely associated with social, situational – i.e. related to certain phases of life – and cultural factors. These factors influence not only the genesis and course of mental disorders but also the perception of symptoms and help-seeking and utilization-of-services behaviour. Severe mental disorders, such as dementia and schizophrenia, are far less influenced by sociocultural factors than are minor mental disturbances. This is probably one

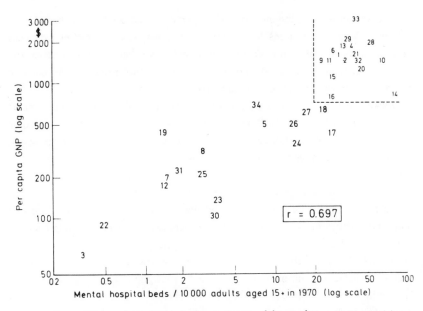

Fig. 1. Ratios of psychiatric beds per 10000 adult population in 34 countries as related to per capita Gross National Product. 1. Australia; 2. Belgium; 3. Burma; 4. Canada; 5. Chile; 6. Denmark; 7. Ghana; 8. Guatemala; 9. France; 10. Finland; 11. Germany, West; 12. Honduras; 13. Iceland; 14. Ireland; 15. Israel; 16. Italy; 17. Jamaica; 18. Japan; 19. Mexico; 20. Netherlands; 21. New Zealand; 22. Pakistan; 23. Philippines; 24. Portugal; 25. Zimbabwe; 26. South Africa; 27. Spain; 28. Sweden; 29. Switzerland; 30. Thailand; 31. Turkey; 32. United Kingdom; 33. United States; 34. Venezuela. Bed ratios are for 1970 (WHO (1962–1978). *World Health Statistics Annual*, Vol. I. WHO, Geneva); GNP data (*Britannica Book of the Year* (1965, 1966, 1967 etc.). *Encyclopaedia Britannica*, Chicago) are from 5 years earlier to allow for development lag. *Source:* Murphy (*94*, P. 24).

of the reasons why transcultural psychiatry has lost more and more ground since Kraepelin's days.

How slight the influence of sociocultural factors is even on the manifestation of psychotic illnesses is shown by the findings of the WHO International Pilot Study of Schizophrenia (*95, 96*) and two later studies (*97, 98*). Starting in 1966 in nine countries differing widely in sociocultural characteristics, the study showed that schizophrenic patients with similar characteristics could be identified in all the nine centres in which the study was conducted, and that the degree of similarity among them could be specified by applying standardized assessment methods ensuring cross-cultural comparability. Furthermore, in all the cultures studied, patients diagnosed as suffering from schizophrenia could be distinguished clearly, in terms of clinical symptoms, from patients with a diagnosis of affective psychosis or another functional mental disorder. It seemed also that a precise and narrow definition of schizophrenia led to quite identical incidence rates in representative first-admission samples across the participating centres (98).

Unlike functional psychoses and mental disorders of organic origin, minor mental disorders vary from culture to culture to a far greater extent. The outcome of the latter disorders and of schizophrenia varies greatly between developing and developed countries, and hence so does their prevalence (95, 96).

Cultural variation in suicide rates

Suicidal acts – including both completed and attempted suicide – are forms of individual behaviour and thus, like other behaviour, subject to judgment by normative and cultural criteria on the part of society.

In some strongly Catholic countries and regions, suicide and attempted suicide used to be liable to punishment by the Church or law, up to as recently as the mid-twentieth century. Among Muslims, too, suicide is regarded as an act of disobedience and resistance to the will of God. In spite of suicides having now ceased to be a social taboo in most countries and its recognition as a behaviour disorder, suicide rates still continue to be lower among Catholics and in mainly Catholic countries than among Protestants. In the Western countries, depressions, of all mental disorders, entail the highest risk for a successfully committed suicide or a suicide attempt of very serious intent (99).

Cultural factors may also cause an elevated suicide rate, as the example of Japan shows. Suicides committed in order to restore lost personal honour are neither related to illness nor are they the result of deviant behaviour in countries where suicide has been considered a moral obligation. Because of its conformity with cultural norms, Durkheim (100) termed this altruistic suicide, as opposed to anomic and egoistic suicide. Even today in countries where suicide used to be a custom or at least more or less tolerated, suicide rates are higher than in cultures that have always disapproved of it.

Culture and alcohol

Since prehistoric times alcohol has been the most important means of conserving beverages. As beverages containing alcohol are very easy to produce and are germ free, they have in many cases replaced infected drinking water. Hence, almost all cultures have been confronted with the problem of alcohol for thousands of years.

According to the status that alcohol has in a culture, we can distinguish three types of culture: abstaining, ambivalent, and permissive (101). Societies in which the prohibition of alcohol and individual abstinence are religiously motivated are

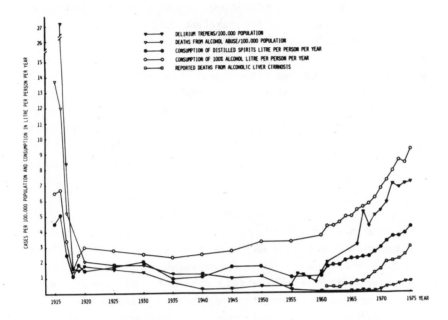

Fig. 2. Correlations among delirium tremens, deaths from chronic alcoholism and liver cirrhosis per 100 000 population, total alcohol consumption in 100% alcohol, and consumption of distilled spirits per person per year. *Source:* Nielsen & Sørensen (*103*).

capable of maintaining the individual risk at a minimum level. In the so-called ambivalent cultures, e.g. in the sphere of Anglo-American Protestantism and the Scandinavian countries, the distribution of alcohol is often subject to temporal and regional restrictions.

The third type comprises the so-called permissive societies, in which alcohol is generally accepted and its consumption is associated with a set of positive values. The use of alcohol is also closely linked with social events: it is regarded as favourable to communication and as a means of strengthening positive social relationships. In these societies it is often not so much drinking as not drinking that runs counter to the expectations of society.

There is also a relationship between social tolerance of alcohol and its availability. It is therefore the right approach to restrict the availability of alcohol as the first step in global preventive programmes (*102*). As the example of Denmark shows, where the availability of alcohol has been restricted by raising the tax on alcoholic liquor proportionally to its level of pure alcohol, preventive programmes have a considerable chance of succeeding. The introduction of the system of taxing alcohol led to a four- to sixfold decrease in per capita consumption, to an eightfold decrease in deaths caused by cirrhosis of the liver, and to a 16-fold drop in the incidence rate of alcoholic delirium (*103*) (see Figure 2). The conclusion that can be drawn from these results is the efficacy of preventive measures that make more difficult the consumption of alcoholic drinks that easily and quickly feed the organism a large amount of alcohol.

The effects of the abolition of existing regulations also serve to illustrate the effectiveness of preventive measures. The lowering of the age limit for the purchase of alcohol from 21 to 18 years in the United States, for example, led, in the year following this legislation, to a rise in alcohol-related accidents by 80%–300% in the age-group 18–21, even though the age restriction had not been strictly observed.

Transcultural aspects of mental illness in old age
The physical risk factors of mental disorders in old age – hypertension, ischaemic heart diseases, and stroke – are altogether rarer in African countries than among black Americans, who are of African descent and should, therefore, not be very different genetically (*104*). An investigation conducted in 30 isolated communities in developing countries has also shown that the rise in blood pressure with age commonly observed in developed countries apparently does not occur in the former. Life-style and salt intake seem to be the main determinants of the differences in risk for hypertension in old age.

Only few findings have as yet been reported on Alzheimer's disease in developing countries. The data available seem to suggest that the disease might be considerably rarer in Black Africa than among black and white Americans (*104*). Provided this difference can be proved and shown not to result from selective mortality of individuals with a higher risk for dementia in African countries, the assumption that it is of environmental rather than genetic origin would gain in credence. Investigations of various populations with a differing risk for hypertension or autoimmune diseases would be necessary to provide clues for causal relationships.

An essential prerequisite for intensification of transnational epidemiological research on and the identification and comparison of risk factors is the development of standardized, transculturally validated assessment methods (*67*).

Social factors and behaviour-related illness
The importance of the family as a model for behaviour
Cultural influences operate largely within social groups, and, in many cases, learning processes within these groups help to establish and maintain self-destructive behaviour. In this context, the role of the family as the very group within which primary socialization takes place is of special importance. For example, Wolin & co-workers (*105*) even use such terms as *transmitter* and *non-*

transmitter families in connection with familial incidence of alcoholism. The model of parental behaviour is of marked importance for the drinking habits of adolescents; parental drinking habits determine not only whether adolescents drink but also what kind of drinks they prefer (*106*).

If adolescents are classified as abstainers, consumers of beer and wine, and regular consumers of spirits, clear relation to the favourite drink of the parents can be observed; this relation exists both in the case of a drinking father and a drinking mother. In the category of abstaining adolescents, the proportion of parents who are abstainers themselves is highest, and that of spirits-consuming parents lowest, when compared with the other two groups, consumers of beer and wine and consumers of spirits. In the category of adolescent consumers of beer and wine, the proportion of abstaining parents is clearly lower, and that of spirits-consuming parents higher than in the category of abstaining adolescents, the favourite parental alcoholic drink being beer or wine. In the group of adolescent consumers of spirits, the proportion of parents also favouring spirits is highest, and that of abstaining parents lowest.

Similar results supporting the hypothesis of parental drinking habits constituting a model for the drinking habits of adolescents were found in investigations of adolescent drug use. Adolescent users of illegal drugs frequently come from families in which one or more persons responsible for the upbringing of children use psychoactive substances (*107–109*). Even if these people generally use only legal drugs, i.e. non-prescription drugs or tranquilizers prescribed by a physician, the children learn to regard drugs as helpful and as a means of solving problems.

Group pressure and peer-group culture

Besides parental reference persons, there are also other factors favouring a drug-oriented socialization. For example, drug-taking within the peer groups exerts a considerable influence on susceptible individuals. It is in the peer group that a favourable attitude toward drugs and the use of drugs is acquired, the prerequisite for a person's decision to start taking drugs. Andrews & Kandell (*110*) were able to show that people starting to take drugs had become acquainted with and adopted the attitudes and ways of thinking of persons already using drugs long before they themselves became drug-users.

The importance of the peer group is also shown by the fact that the number of adolescents who start to experiment with drugs on their own initiative is irrelevantly low, whereas 90% of all users were found to have had their first contacts with drugs in the company of friends and peers (*108*). The use of drugs – among adolescents in particular – is a group-related phenomenon, the initial diffusion taking place within small, clearly definable groups confined to certain areas.

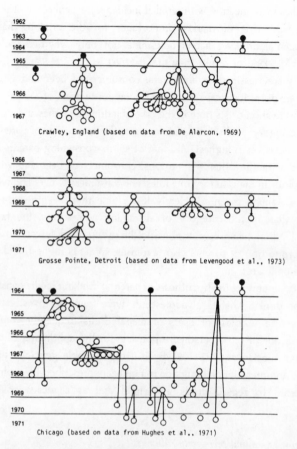

Fig. 3. Microdiffusion of drug abuse: epidemic diffusion of heroin dependence in Crawley, Grosse Pointe and Chicago (based on data from De Alarcon (*111*), Levengood *et al.* (*112*) and Hughes *et al.* (*113*)). *Source:* Welz, R., Niedermaier, C. (1983). Diffusionstheorie der Ausbreitung des Drogenkonsums. In: D. J. Lettieri & R. Welz (eds.) *Drogenabhängigkeit. Ursachen und Verlaufsformen. Ein Handbuch.* 1. Psychologie Verlags-Union Beltz: 2. Munich, Weinheim, pp. 235–245.

The spread of a psychological disorder: microdiffusion of drug abuse as an illustration
The ensuing diffusion of drug abuse, initiated within small groups, has been studied, among others, by Alarcon (*111*), in the English town of Crawley; by Levengood, Lowinger, & Schoof (*112*), in Grosse Pointe, a community in the vicinity of Detroit, Michigan; and by Hughes & co-workers (*113*, *114*), in Chicago. The authors interviewed former drug addicts and their drug-using and non-drug-using friends. With the help of these key informants, traced down in interviews, the channels of diffusion into formerly drug-free areas were determined.

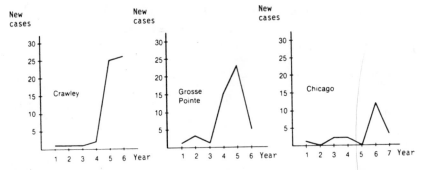

Fig. 4. Epidemic diffusion of drug abuse (based on data from Chambers & Hunt (*116*)). *Source:* Welz, R. Niedermaier, C. (1983). Diffusionstheorie der Ausbreitung des Drogenkonsums. In: D. J. Lettieri & R. Welz (eds.) *Drogenabhängigkeit. Ursachen und Verlaufsformen. Ein Handbuch.* Psychologie Verlags-Union Beltz: Munich, Weinheim, pp. 235–245.

Figure 3 illustrates the spread of drug abuse from individual to individual. It also shows that there are isolated and comparatively isolated people who pass the technique of heroin use to no other, or to only one other person, and users who introduce several persons to drug abuse. On the basis of the diagrams in Figure 3, Welz (*115*) has worked out a more differentiated and more generally applicable description of the diffusion channels by calculating the annual number of new drug-takers; the number of drug-users with no, one, two, etc. imitators; and the time it takes for already active users to produce imitators.

The curve in Figure 4 illustrating the epidemic diffusion of drug abuse into formerly drug-free areas shows that, in the initial period, the number of new drug-users hardly changes, or increases only slightly, but experiences a steep increase between the third and sixth year, and then increases only slightly or even falls thereafter. Thus, the spread of drug abuse conforms largely to the s-shaped curve characteristic of the diffusion process described by Rogers & Shoemaker (*117*). This course of the diffusion process is closely linked to the growing influence of those who have already accepted and adopted the new behaviour.

As Table 4 shows, there have to be several active users if the behaviour is to spread. The majority of active users produce no imitators, some users only one or two, and only very few introduce several individuals to drug-taking. The result is the same whether we consider the diagrams in Figure 4 separately or add up the values of all three diagrams. The diffusion of drug dependence thus hinges on the activity of only a few individuals.

Since the production of several imitators is unlikely, the implications for a rapid epidemic increase are that users with several imitators each succeed one another in a comparatively short period of time. In the initial phase of diffusion within small

Table 4. *Distribution of drug users with 0, 1, 2, ... n imitators*

| Area of study | Number of followers | | | | | | |
	0	1	2	3	4	5	6 and more
Crawley 1962–1967	30	10	4	–	3	1	1
Grosse Pointe 1966–1971	25	8	3	2	–	2	–
Chicago 1964–1971	35	11	7	2	–	1	1
Total	90	29	14	3	–	4	2

Source: Welz (*115*), p. 132.

local groups, too, a relatively high influx of users from outside these groups is necessary, because many of these users produce no imitators; others, only one; and only a few, several imitators. Still another finding was that, in 90% of cases, the transmission of the drug-taking habit had been completed within the first year or in the course of the second year.

The findings seem plausible considering the fact that it is the new user who has the most influence on other potential users. In a few months' time he will have become dependent and will begin to suffer from the after-effects of that dependence. Not only does he lose his credibility and attractiveness but his social reference groups begin to change. He will leave school or his job, descend in the social scale, and his circle of friends will change (*116*). In other words, as a result of these successive changes due to his addiction, the initiator loses his formerly contagious social qualities. It is not the users characterized by social decline and the physical effects of drug-taking who act as initiators, but the users of the early phase, who will have lost their contagious features in the course of the first year.

The most important findings on the diffusion of drug-taking within small groups can be summed up as follows: the diffusion of drug abuse is a group-related phenomenon, and the users generally describe the initiators as friends or important reference persons. Hence, each user has as many imitators as there are members in the group he has entered or of which he is a member. As noted above, all users are most likely to transmit the drug-taking habit at the beginning of their drug career, usually in the first year. The consumption of heroin experiences an epidemic diffusion provided a susceptible group comes into contact with several contagious users. The diffusion comes to a halt when all potential imitators have been reached or when the users are not capable of reaching all susceptible persons, in which case they may seek contact with other groups, enter them, and in this way begin to undergo changes in spatial terms as well.

Social disintegration

Faris & Dunham (*118*) were the first to show that the social environment people live in may influence the frequency of mental disorder. They found that first consultations because of schizophrenia were more frequent in downtown Chicago than in the more affluent suburban residential areas. Studies on drug abuse (*119, 120*) or suicidal behaviour (*121–125*) have almost unanimously revealed that drug abuse and suicidal behaviour prevail in downtown areas characterized by high rates of mobility and fluctuation, a high percentage of single and elderly residents, and high crime and morbidity rates.

In order to obtain more detailed information on the structure of neighbourhoods with high rates of attempted suicide, Welz (*126*) conducted a cluster analysis. He collected data on all inhabitants of the medium-sized German city of Mannheim who had attempted suicide over a ten-year period. The ecological study and the cluster analysis were based on 78 enumeration districts. The analysis yielded four homogeneous groups comprising 14, 45, 9, and 10 small-scale urban areas, respectively. The findings on area characteristics determined by cluster analysis and the rate of attempted suicide over a ten-year period are presented in Table 5.

In total, several types of area clusters were found to characterize four different types of social structure:

- The first cluster describes a high-standard area with a low rate of blue-collar workers and a high rate of social disintegration, i.e. high rates for divorced persons and one-person households, disrupted families, and a high proportion of persons per housing unit.
- The second and third clusters describe a middle-class setting and a working-class area.
- The fourth cluster can be characterized as a low-standard, working-class area with the characteristics of social disintegration.

In both the middle-class and the working-class areas the rate of attempted suicide was below the average rate for Mannheim as a whole. Two homogeneous suicidal areas were found in which both social anomia and social disintegration were high. As the two 'suicidal areas' differed in terms of their social status, a low level of social integration proved to be a very strong variable explaining the urban distribution of some behavioural disorders.

The high incidence of attempted suicide in both working-class and upper-middle-class areas characterized by social disintegration points to factors influencing social integration and life within social groups.

Social status and mental health

Social status and social class are among the main factors influencing mental health and life expectancy. Hence, it is not surprising that of the great variety of potential ecological impacts on mental health, the association between socio-economic status and risk of mental illness has received most attention from researchers.

Brugger (*127, 128*) in the course of enumerative surveys of mental illness, was among the first to report indications of a high frequency of schizophrenia in low occupational groups in Thuringen and Upper Bavaria. Later, Tietze, Lemkau & Cooper (*129*) and Hollingshead & Redlich (*130*), in the United States, found a correlation between low occupational status and high first-admission rates for schizophrenia. Dohrenwend & Dohrenwend (*22*), in a literature review, came to the conclusion that the high first-admission rates in the lower classes was a largely, even if not absolutely, consistent finding.

Ecological studies – starting with the classic study by Faris & Dunham (*118*) in Chicago – have also shown first-admission rates for schizophrenia to be highest in districts characterized by the lowest standard of housing and the lowest socioeconomic status. The concentration of high first-admission rates in areas of low socioeconomic status has also proved to be a fairly consistent finding of numerous comparable studies, conducted in Kansas City and St. Louis, Missouri (*131*), Rochester, New York (*132*), Detroit, Michigan (*133*), Oslo, Norway (*134*), Bristol, England (*51*), Dublin, Ireland (*135*), and Mannheim, FRG (*136*), to mention a few examples.

To sum up the findings, most schizophrenic patients come from residential areas of low social status within large cities and belong to the lower socioeconomic classes. Similar results were also found concerning the distribution of dementia in urban areas (*118*), mental disorder in old age (*68*), and mental retardation (*137*). This, however, does not apply to medium-sized or small towns of homogeneous socioecological structures in Norway (*138*) – and probably also in many other countries.

Studies on the use of narcotics in Chicago (*139*), Manhattan (*119*), and on the Lower East side of Manhattan, New York, and, to some extent, the investigations carried out in Mannheim (*116*) have also revealed a close association between low social class, economic deprivation, and familial disintegration. Similarly, certain subgroups of alcoholics (*140, 141*) and suicides or suicide attempters (*122, 142*) come from the lower classes and residential areas of low social status.

The incidence of certain categories of mental disorder in the lowest stratum is a fairly consistent finding, but membership in the lowest social class is too imprecise a variable to explain the association. The relationship between poor socioeconomic status and a high risk for mental morbidity may also result from social selection or drift processes; certain people descend in the social scale because

Table 5. *Area characteristics as determined by cluster analysis*

Ecological variable	Cluster I	Cluster II	Cluster III	Cluster IV	Mannheim total
Blue-collar workers	32.68	46.67	64.12	61.72	48.11
Housing units w/o bathrooms	14.62	15.99	9.23	24.97	16.11
65 and over	14.69	11.46	3.18	5.46	10.32
Youth dependency	35.90	45.30	30.18	75.95	46.18
Persons/housing unit	19.05	7.95	7.77	16.53	11.18
Divorced	4.12	2.21	1.09	2.24	2.43
Disrupted families	11.14	7.21	2.98	14.60	8.37
Single females with children	2.90	2.08	0.99	4.86	2.46
1-person households	42.38	30.61	28.87	21.06	31.22
Mobility	414.67	327.66	618.74	485.77	396.91
Tenants	87.67	64.09	78.98	81.03	72.21
Attempted suicide	12.64	8.44	6.27	14.33	9.76

of premorbid personality traits or psychological impairment and wind up in areas of low socioeconomic status.

It should also be asked which characteristics correlating with a low social class actually account for this relationship and influence mental health and morbidity risk. If belonging to a lower social class proves to correlate with variables increasing the risk of mental disorder, the global relationship between social class and incidence of mental disorder has to be interpreted as an indirect relationship geared to other variables, such as a higher risk of losing one's job, lack of knowledge of the consequences of certain behaviour detrimental to mental health, lack of effective coping styles, or insufficient health or help-seeking behaviour.

Social causation or social selection in schizophrenia

High first-admission rates for schizophrenia in substandard living areas of low social status are a consistent finding in psychiatric epidemiological studies. Thus, the question arises whether unfavourable socioeconomic conditions of ecological variables contribute to the causation of schizophrenia (the breeder hypothesis), or whether only intra- or intergenerational selection leads to an increase in schizophrenia among the lower classes and in poor living areas.

Referring to the findings of Tietze and co-workers (*129*), Hollingshead & Redlich (*130*), Clausen & Kohn (*143*), Srole and associates (*40*), Goldberg & Morrison (*144*), and Turner & Wagenfeld (*145*), Häfner (*146, 147*) has discussed the suggestion that the relation between social class and mental disorder does not depend solely on intervening variables, but is the result of social selection processes. Although the findings of the studies investigating intergeneration mobility among schizophrenics (with regard to the selection hypothesis) are not consistent, they predominantly show that lack of social success and downward mobility in families afflicted by schizophrenia seem to be a major factor and need to be taken into account when explaining the higher incidence rates in the lowest social classes.

Tietze & associates (*129*), Hollingshead & Redlich (*130*), and Clausen & Kohn (*143*) found, for example, that in most cases fathers belonged to the same social class as their schizophrenic sons. The studies by Srole & co-workers (*40*), Goldberg & Morrison (*144*), Turner & Wagenfeld (*145*), and Goodman & colleagues (*148*) also contain indications of low social achievement among schizophrenics that in some cases can be observed even in succeeding generations. In the Midtown Manhattan Study, Srole & co-workers (*40*) found that among the fathers of psychotics, the distribution across social classes was analogous to but less pronounced than in the index cases. Turner & Wagenfeld (*145*), basing their study on a sample of male schizophrenics included in the case register of Monroe County, New York, observed that approximately three times as many schizophrenics, but still more than twice as many of their fathers, as expected from the average figures for the total population, belonged to the lower social classes.

Further evidence in support of the selection hypothesis is provided by an investigation, based on the Norwegian case register, of the relation between morbidity rates for schizophrenia and migration. Dalgard (*149*) and Odegard (*138*) found significantly lower first-admission rates for schizophrenia in migrants from rural to urban areas and from large cities to suburbs; the frequency of first admissions was greater among migrants from urban to rural areas.

The long-term changes in first-admission rates for schizophrenia across various occupational groups from 1926 to 1965 (*138*) provide further evidence of the selection hypothesis. In Norway the occupational groups with unusually high first-admission rates for schizophrenia (seamen and farm workers) show a sharp decline in employment. Odegard (*138*) demonstrated this process using as an example female domestic servants, an occupation that today has almost died out in Norway. The exceptionally high first-admission rates for schizophrenia in this occupational group contrasted with significantly lower rates for single housewives without outside occupation, a group that differed very little with respect to their situation in life and work. From this Odegard concluded that only people who avoid changing to more successful occupations because of their disability remain in occupations that are dying out and offer little chances for advancement. They are joined by newly disabled people from other occupational groups for whom the lower threshold of qualification makes it possible to get employment.

Odegard concluded that the selection hypothesis accounted for his findings on geographic migration. Premorbid personality traits, lack of social relationships, and, particularly, lack of occupational success make it easier to decide to leave home and occupation. This explains why in migration streams connected with social ascent there are relatively few people with a predisposition to schizophrenia, whereas in migration streams of those with little social success there are relatively many (*147*).

Clear evidence of social selection processes can also be found in alcoholism. Dietrich & Herle (*140*) compared the occupational skills acquired and practiced by alcoholics with the occupations of their fathers at hospitalization. The study revealed that the inter- and intrageneration mobility among alcoholics was characterized by social decline. Social decline was also linked with moving to low-standard housing areas (*141*).

These findings supporting the selection hypothesis are backed by the results of studies conducted on twins and siblings. Controlled investigations on the offspring of schizophrenic parents, discordant identical twins, or schizophrenics and their disorder-free siblings indicate that even before onset of the illness, behavioural differences that seem to influence social success can be observed. As early as in elementary school, future schizophrenics lag substantially behind their brothers and sisters in terms of IQ and school performance (*150*). Moreover, compared with their brothers and sisters or co-twins, the schizophrenics-to-be have fewer social contacts, are less independent or dominant, exhibiting, more often, dependency relationships and unspecific symptoms (*151*). In conformity with the findings of epidemiological twin studies and a Danish study on adopted offspring (*152–157*), we may assume that psychological changes weaken the chances of social success of persons with a predisposition to schizophrenia long before the psychosis manifests itself.

Services utilization and help-seeking behaviour

The factors determining help-seeking behaviour and readiness to utilize professional medical or psychiatric services clearly correlate with social class. The relation between family income and number of consultations in the United States, where people have to pay for medical services, has often been described (*158*). But the relationship is more complex than it seems to be at first glance. In spite of a substantial reduction in consultation fees or their complete abolition, as in Sweden and Great Britain (*159*), there seems still to be an association between social class and frequency of consultation.

In addition to a possible influence of family income, Suchman (*160*) was able to demonstrate differences in attitudes toward illness as further reasons for physician-averse behaviour in the lower classes in the United States. He found that members of the lower classes had less information and knowledge about illnesses and their treatment and were highly sceptical of health care services. Furthermore, members of the lower classes exhibited an equally averse attitude toward another very important variable of illness behaviour, i.e. acceptance of their illness and of the ensuing dependence on physicians: they were less willing to accept the fact of being ill and to rely on the services of physicians than were members of the higher social classes.

Reimann & Häfner (*161*) were able to show, for mental disorders related to old age (over 60 years), that a higher socioeconomic status correlated with a higher frequency of consulting psychiatrists in free practice at an earlier stage of illness, whereas a lower socioeconomic status correlated with a higher rate of admissions to the state psychiatric hospital at a more advanced stage of illness.

If an analysis of the factors determining services utilization and help-seeking behaviour is to take account of attitudes toward health services and illness as such, allowance must be made for the special situation of the mentally ill. In a study of the influence of social attitudes favourable or unfavourable to consultation of medical services, Moeller (*162*) stressed the special case of the mentally ill, who may display a far stronger aversion than do physically ill people toward consulting physicians when lack of self-confidence and fear of meeting other people, on the one hand, and a kind of indifference, on the other, are among the symptoms of the illness.

The influence of stressful life events on morbidity risk

The influence of stressful life events on morbidity risk has been demonstrated for some physical illnesses (*163*) and almost all mental disorders. The relative risk associated with stressful life events varies according to the type of mental disorder. It is particularly high in depression and still more marked in attempted suicide (*164*). Persons who attempted suicide mentioned more stressful life events during the six months before their attempt than did depressive persons or healthy controls (for the same period). Among those who had attempted suicide, a descriptive analysis of the temporal distribution of stressful life events showed a marked concentration of such events in the month preceding the attempt. For persons suffering from acute depression, the rate of such events had increased slightly in the two months before hospitalization; the rate for the controls had remained constant for the preceding six months.

As Kuhnt, Kleff, & Welz (*165*) have shown, the risk associated with stressful life events varies according to the subgroups of suicidal persons. By means of the Suicide Intention and Seriousness Scale (SISS) developed by Häfner & co-workers (*99*), Kuhnt and associates distinguished two groups with suicidal behaviour. A comparison of the distribution of stressful life events over the previous six months for both groups led to the conclusion that the group characterized by less serious suicide attempts had had more stressful life events. Particularly frequent mention was made of life events involving personal relationships and changes in economic status, occupation, and place of work.

Unemployment is of particular importance. In their classic study of the unemployed in Marienthal, Austria, Jahoda, Lazarsfeld, & Zeisel (*166*) were among the first to point out the consequences of unemployment for mental health. Marienthal is a small community near Vienna. At the time of the study, around the turn of the year 1931–32, the population of the community totalled 1486. Before the outbreak of the Depression of 1929, a textile factory offered sufficient employment, and layoffs were fairly rare. Anybody who settled in Marienthal found work, even for his wife and children, in the factory. As a consequence of the central role the factory played in offering jobs, its closing in 1929 led to a situation in which almost the entire population suddenly found itself out of work. Jahoda & co-workers observed resignation, despair, apathy, alcohol problems, and depression in 77% of the unemployed. Characteristic of the collective response of despair, resignation, and depression were also a decline and slackening-off of almost all social activities. Despite the fact that, being unemployed, people had more time to read, the number of cost-free loans of books by the public library fell by 48.7%;

subscriptions for the workers' newspaper decreased by 60%; and membership in the local sports club dropped by 52% despite reduced membership fees for the unemployed.

A generation later, Cobb & Gore (167–169) studied the physical and mental health of workers in connection with factory closures. Of the 22 indicators of mental health under examination, 15 showed significant changes, depending on the length of unemployment. This applied especially when social support was used as a control variable. Workers with sufficient social support within their families and with more extensive social relationships exhibited milder symptoms of depression, although they had been unemployed an equally long time. With regard to physical illness as well (the most distinct relationship was found between stress and diseases of the joints), extensive social support proved to have a protective effect (167). Of those with poor social support, 41% exhibited mental disorders, compared with 4% of those with excellent and 12% of those with adequate social support resources.

In addition to occupational problems, which are more common in the lower classes, Pearlin & Schooler (170) regard ineffective coping mechanisms as another factor in higher rates of mental morbidity among those classes. People belonging to the lower classes have less effective coping resources – e.g. personality traits such as self-esteem and a sense of master – than do members of the middle or higher classes. Indeed, members of the lower classes referred to their low self-esteem and said they had hardly any influence on the course of their lives.

Migration and social changes

Both migration and social change confront people with a need to adjust to new conditions. Migration can be motivated by positive expectations of social advancement, better working conditions, and higher income; but migrants are expected to adjust to a new culture and to the social norms of the host country. Enculturation and acculturation, together with failure to achieve the anticipated rapid social success, constitute three risk factors to which migrants, most of whom come from the lower social classes, are exposed. Social change involving changes in, and a gradual weakening of, behaviour-stabilizing norms without an immediate replacement by new ones also produces a period characterized by uncertainty and disruptions in social relationships.

It is a common feature of immigrant groups, such as the Norwegians in Minnesota (171) or the Hungarians in Norway (172), that they have usually left behind their families and the social networks within which they had grown up in order to go and live in an unfamiliar culture. In migratory workers, leaving their home countries voluntarily for a certain time, the separation seems to cause less strain or burden than in political refugees. Häfner, Moschel, & Özek (173), assisted by a Turkish psychiatrist, found, in a prospective study, that 75% of a group of

Turkish workers, of more or less homogeneous composition in terms of origin, age, sex, and occupational status and examined prospectively, displayed no signs of mental disorder two weeks and three months after their arrival in the Federal Republic of Germany. Pflanz, Hasenkopf, & Costas (174), examining a group of Greek workers, and Binder & Simoes (175), examining Portuguese workers in Switzerland, also found lower incidence rates of psychosomatic disorders and mental disturbances, including depressive syndromes, in the foreign workers than in control groups of workers in their native countries.

The case-register study on psychiatric morbidity among foreign workers in Mannheim, conducted by Häfner (176), underlines the extraordinary importance of the selection hypothesis. In the period of investigation – 1 January 1974 to 31 December 1978 – about 13% of the Mannheim population were foreigners. The age composition of the foreign workers showed an overrepresentation of younger age groups, thus differing markedly from the German population. Consequently, the rates for mental morbidity among the foreign workers were correspondingly lower. When corrected for age, the rates for treated schizophrenic episodes (a comparison of first-admission rates was not feasible because of their low number) were still significantly lower than those for the German population. The lowest rates were found among Turks, and, in comparison with the native population, the rates among Italians were slightly reduced. Yugoslavs and other foreigners, among whom refugees predominated, did not differ significantly from the native population.

The rates for alcohol-related diseases and organic brain syndromes were similar to the frequency of schizophrenia, lower among the immigrants than in the native population, whereas the rates for affective psychoses and neurotic and psycho-somatic disorders did not differ markedly between the foreign groups and the German population.

Because of the low rates found by Pflanz & co-workers (174) for Greek workers and by Binder & Simoes (175) for Portuguese immigrants, Häfner has stressed that selective factors may have an influence on the low frequency of mental disorder reported among immigrants. He assumes that both the decision to go abroad to work and the chances of passing a medical screening before emigration would have been influenced by an early onset of chronic disease or by premorbid personality abnormalities. Medical examination of Turkish workers by the German labour administration was most severe.

The reason for higher morbidity rates for women among foreign workers may be that they contribute less to the decision to emigrate and that they undergo a less thorough examination.

Unlike emigrant groups, foreign workers represent a positive selection with regard to predisposition to schizophrenia and other long-term mental disorders. Thus, in the relatively poorer regions from which large proportions of the healthy, able-to-work population emigrate, mainly those who are old or suffering from chronic mental or physical disorders remain behind. This may result not only in an unhealthy population structure but also in a relative increase in the morbidity rates for schizophrenia.

Trends in morbidity

Schizophrenia

In contrast to the considerable variation in the frequency of deviant behaviour and the related health risks, the risk of schizophrenia seems not to have undergone any great changes in the last few decades (117). Under the title *Psychosis and Civilization*, Goldhamer & Marshall (178) compared first-admission rates for 'psychoses of the early and medium adult life' by five-year periods for 1840–85 and 1940. Over the period of 100 years, the crude first-admission rates rose from about 40/100 000 to about 70/100 000, the highest rise occurring mainly between 1845 and 1885. After analysing various factors, these authors concluded that a long-term increase in the risk of falling ill with schizophrenia could be excluded.

The trend in Goldhamer & Marshall's study has been confirmed in several others, e.g. by Dunham (179), examining first admissions for schizophrenia to the psychiatric hospitals of seven states of the United States between 1910 and 1950; and by Kramer, von Korff & Kessler (180) and by Torrey (181), using data from national statistics on first admissions for schizophrenia to psychiatric hospitals throughout the United States between 1922 and 1960. Torrey, however, gave the same data an inverse interpretation. In his publication, similarly entitled *Schizophrenia and Civilization*, he attempted to prove that with the advance of civilization, the risk of schizophrenia had increased, particularly in the nineteenth century. Eaton (182), who ascertained the rates for first admissions for schizophrenia to the mental hospitals of Massachusetts for a further 15 years, also concluded that his and Goldhamer & Marshall's data might be interpreted as indicating a threefold rise in the incidence rates over a period of 115 years.

The only conclusion that can be drawn from the above data, in contrast to Torrey's and Eaton's interpretations, is that the incidence rates for schizophrenia, in the populations in which they have been studied, have neither increased nor decreased sharply. More precise interpretations would require consideration of changes in the age structure of the population over the period under study, of the comparability of the diagnoses, and of the rate of utilization of services, i.e. the proportion of patients who actually consulted psychiatric services when the illness first appeared.

The only study focusing on changing case definitions, a factor of decisive importance when using morbidity data (particularly from the nineteenth century), is that conducted by Krupinski & Alexander (183) on admissions to mental hospitals in Victoria, Australia, over the period 1848–1978. These investigators

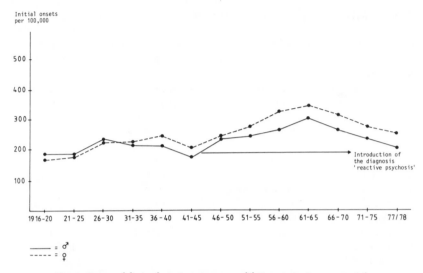

Fig. 5. Rates of first admissions per year (lifetime expectancy rates) for schizophrenia in Norway from 1919 to 1978 (based on data collected by Astrup[2]). *Source:* Häfner (*177*).

found that the admission rates for functional psychoses remained unaltered until the tasks of the mental health services were expanded in 1952. Among the functional psychoses, manias decreased continuously, from approximately 70% in 1848 to about 0% in 1950. Over the same period, admissions with the diagnosis 'delusional insanity', later 'dementia praecox', later 'schizophrenia', increased, from about 25% to about 80%.

Krupinski & Alexander diagnosed samples of 100 admissions each from several periods retrospectively according to DSM-III criteria. They found that from 1848 to the present time, in a decreasing sequence, about 80%, 60%, 40%, and finally, 0% of the cases originally diagnosed as 'manias' and some 30% of those diagnosed as 'melancholias' in the last century would today be classified as schizophrenias. If the quantitative impact of this process of change, which Krupinski & Alexander proved by historical analysis of the concepts of mental illness for a period extending from Esquirol's, through Griesinger's, to Kraepelin's days, is taken into account, a stable course of admission rates for schizophrenia – by DSM-III criteria – for over 130 years emerges.

On the basis of the data provided by the Norwegian case register, including all Norwegians who have received inpatient treatment since 1917, Astrup[2] determined the incidence rates for schizophrenia by investigating five-year age groups in relation to the population of the same five birth years from the Norwegian population. The incidence rates for schizophrenia, thus controlled for age, had undergone only slight changes over more than 50 years (see Figure 5) (*177*).

Table 6. *Incidence rates for schizophrenia from psychiatric case registers*

(Including data from Case Registers in Europe, USA plus Australia for comparison)
Incidence rate = first contacts with a psychiatric case register per year and per 1000
total population.

Place	Author	Year	Rate/1000
Norway	Astrup[a] Note 2	1926–30	0.23[a]
Norway	Astrup Note 2	1977/78	0.24[a]
Iceland	Helgason (185)	1966/67	0.27
Camberwell, UK	Wing & Fryers (186)	1976	0.13
Salford, UK	Wing & Fryers (186)	1976	0.13
Denmark	Munk-Jörgensen (187)	1972	0.12
Victoria, Australia	Krupinski[g]	1978	0.16
Netherlands	Giel et al. (188)	1978/79	0.11[b]
South Verona, Italy	Tansella et al. (189)	1983	0.08[c,d]
Maryland, USA	Warthen et al. (190)	1963	0.50
Mannheim, FRG	Häfner & Reimann (136)	1965	0.54
Mannheim, FRG	Häfner et al. Note 4	1974–80[f]	0.59
Rochester, USA	Babigian (191)	1970	0.69
Upper Bavaria, FRG	Dilling et al. (192)	1975	0.48

[a] 'Lifetime expectancy rate', hospitalized cases only, schizophrenia and 'reactive psychoses'.
[b] Including ICD 297.0–297.9; 298.3–298.9.
[c] Rate for first-ever contacts.
[d] Rate for schizophrenia and schizophrenialike psychoses.
[e] Survey based on comparable sources of data collection.
[f] Data from the Cumulative Psychiatric Case Register of the Central Institute of Mental
Health, Mannheim (ICD-8: 295, 297, 298.3); rate for population aged 12–59 and a broad
definition of diagnosis; rate for a restrictive definition: 0.31/1000.
[g] Personal communication, 1984.

Sources: Häfner & an der Heiden (147), Eaton (193) and Munk-Jörgensen (187).

For the purpose of comparison, Figure 5 also indicates age-standardized rates for
an initial diagnosis of dementia in males. Since we can agree with Odegard (138)
that the diagnosis of schizophrenia has become comparatively reliable and stable
in Norway since the introduction of the diagnostic system developed by Kraepelin
(see also Klug [184]), we can conclude, at least for Victoria, Australia, and Norway,
that, despite substantial changes in living conditions, the actual prevalence of
schizophrenia remained unchanged in the period studied.

More recent case-register studies (see Table 6), which have revealed markedly
low variations in incidence rates (between 0.11 and 0.69 per 100000 of the
population), do not support the theory of the dependence of incidence rates on
cultural developments or long-term social change.

Other mental disorders

The question whether mental disorders of such high frequency as depressive illnesses have decreased or increased remains unanswered. In the course of their study conducted in two phases (1947–62 and 1963–72), Hagnell & Öjesjö[3] found a clear increase in the age-controlled risk or milder depressive states in the population of about 5000 of the community of Lundby, in Southern Sweden. But since the diagnosis of less severe forms of depression is affected by self-definitions and imprecise diagnostic concepts, and since the diagnoses were established in free psychiatric interviews in both phases of the study, the assumed increase cannot yet be regarded as proven.

Häfner (*177*), in his analysis, states that, in milder mental disorders, the increase in seeking medical care is due mainly to new treatment methods and to the great expansion of psychiatric and psychotherapeutic services in most industrial countries, in which a *Zeitgeist* characterized by a transition from an understanding of life determined by natural science to a more 'psychological' interpretation forms the background.

Conclusions

The frequency, severity, first onset, distribution, course, and outcome of mental illness may be subject to environmental factors. These factors range from global, culture-related influences to community-related factors and those stemming from the social network of family and other social groups, such as the peer group and the neighbourhood (see also H. Häfner & R. Welz, 'Social networks and mental disorder', in this volume). However, not all mental disorders are equally subject to environmental variability.

A good example of epidemiological research on the social and social-psychological influences on the genesis and diffusion of widespread mental illness is provided by studies on drug and alcohol abuse. In this area it has even been possible to translate some of the research results into effective programmes. On the other hand, for schizophrenia the results obtained indicate that the influence of social factors upon the risk of falling ill and the influence of the uneven distribution over social classes on the frequency of initial onset have to be assessed more conservatively. The only slight variation in the frequency of schizophrenia over the last 50–100 years is noteworthy.

Besides the mental status associated with life events, individual coping styles, and social-support resources, all of which play an important role in minor mental disorders, imitation and processes of social influence have a decisive impact on suicidal behaviour and on the spread of drug and alcohol abuse.

In the course of rapid changes in living conditions, new factors detrimental to mental health have arisen. There have also been changes in the demographic structure of most populations, marked by an increased proportion of the elderly, with a concomitant increase in both physical and mental disorders. In all age groups, but especially among the elderly, physical and mental illness often interact, and alleviation of physical illness frequently leads also to improved mental health – and vice versa. Increased research on the life situation of the elderly and on the interaction between physical and mental health at all ages is needed, so that successful preventive measures and effective treatment can be developed.

Notes

1. N. Sartorius, A. Jablensky, A. Korten, G. Ernberg, M. Anker, J. E. Cooper, & R. Day, Early manifestations and first contact incidence of schizophrenia in different cultures *Psychological Medicine*, 1986, 16: 909–928.
2. C. Astrup, The increase of mental disorders. Unpublished manuscript from the National Case Register of Mental Disorders, Gaustad Hospital, Oslo, Norway, 1982.
3. O. Hagnell & J. Öjesjö, Lundby, 15–25 years later. Paper presented at the World Psychiatric Association Symposium 'Social causes of mental disorders', Opatja, Yugoslavia, September 1975.
4. Häfner, H., Riecher, A., Maurer, K. & Löffler, W. Sex-specific differences in age at first onset of schizophrenic disorders. Poster presented at the '4th Bi-Ennal Winter Workshop on Schizophrenia', Badgastein, Austria, 24–29 January, 1988.

References

1. Reed, T. E., Kalant, H., Gibbins, R. J., Kapur, B. M., & Rankin, J. D. Alcohol and acetaldehyde metabolism in Caucasians, Chinese and Amerinds. *Canadian Medical Association Journal*, **115**, 851–55 (1976).
2. Wartburg, J. P. v., Papenburg, H., & Aebi, H. An atypical human alcohol dehydrogenase. *Canadian Journal of Biochemistry*, **43**, 889 (1965).
3. Propping, P. Genetische Aspekte des Alkoholismus. In H. Häfner & R. Welz (Eds.), *Drogenabhängigkeit und Alkoholismus*, Köln., Rheinland Verlag, 1981. Vol. 7, pp. 95–106.
4. Goedde, H. S., Harada, S., & Agarwal, D. P. Racial differences in alcohol sensitivity: A new hypothesis. *Human Genetics*, **51**, 331–34 (1979).
5. Inoue, K., Fukunaga, M., & Yamasawa, K. Correlation betwen human erythrocyte aldehyde dehydrogenase activity and sensitivity to alcohol. *Pharmacology, Biochemistry, and Behavior*, **13**, 295–97 (1980).
6. Propping, P. Genetische Aspekte des Alkoholismus. In D. J. Lettieri & R. Welz (Eds.), *Drogenabhängigkeit–Ursachen und Verlaufsformen. Ein Handbuch*. Weinheim, Beltz, 1983. Pp. 311–22.
7. Robins, L. N. *A follow-up of Vietnam drug users*. Washington, DC, U.S. Government Printing Office, 1973.
8. Robins, L. N. Theorie der Drogenauffälligkeit bei Jugendlichen. In D. J. Lettieri &

R. Welz (Eds.), *Drogenabhängigkeit–Ursachen und Verlaufsformen. Ein Handbuch.* Weinheim, Beltz, 1983. Pp. 225–34.

9. Shepherd, M., Cooper, B., Brown, A. C., & Kalton, G. W. *Psychiatric illness in general practice.* London, Oxford University Press.

10. Dilling, H., Weyerer, S., & Enders, J. Patienten mit psychischen Störungen in der Allgemeinpraxis und ihre psychiatrische Überweisungsbedürftigkeit. In H. Häfner (Ed.), *Psychiatrische Epidemiologie.* Berlin, Springer, 1978. Pp. 135–60.

11. Zintl-Wiegand, A., & Cooper, B. Psychische Erkrankungen in der Allgemeinpraxis: Eine Untersuchung in Mannheim. *Nervenarzt*, **50**, 352–59 (1979).

12. Strotzka, H. *Kleinburg–Eine socialpsychiatrische Feldstudie.* Wien, Österreichischer Bundesverlag, 1969.

13. Cooper, B., & Morgan, H. G. *Epidemiological psychiatry.* Springfield, IL, Charles C. Thomas, 1973.

14. Wing, J. K., & Fryers, T. *Psychiatric services in Camberwell and Salford. Statistics from the Camberwell and Salford psychiatric registers, 1964–1974.* London, MRC Social Psychiatric Unit, and Manchester, Department of Community Medicine, University of Manchester, 1976.

15. Baldwin, J. A. *The mental hospital in the psychiatric service. A case-register study.* London, Oxford University Press, 1971.

16. Hall, D. J., Robertson, N. C., & Eason, R. J. (Eds.) *Proceedings of the Conference on Psychiatric Case Registers at the University of Aberdeen, March 1973.* London, Her Majesty's Stationery Office, 1974.

17. Wing, J. K., & Hailey, A. M. *Evaluating a community psychiatric service.* London, Oxford University Press, 1972.

18. Häfner, H., Moschel, G., & Sartorius, N. (Eds.) *Mental health in the elderly. A review of the present state of research.* Berlin, Heidelberg, New York, Tokyo, Springer, 1986.

19. Häfner, H., & Klug, J. The impact of an expanding community mental health service on patterns of bed usage: Evaluation of a four-year period of implementation. *Psychological Medicine*, **12**, 177–90 (1982).

20. Brunetti, P. M. Rural Vaucluse. Two surveys on the prevalence of mental disorder. Summary of data. *Acta Psychiatrica Scandinavica*, **51**, Suppl. 263, pp. 12–15 (1975).

21. Leighton, D. C., Harding, J. S., Mackline, D. B., Macmillan, A. M., & Leighton, A. H. *The Stirling County Study III: The character of danger.* New York, Basic Books, 1963.

22. Dohrenwend, B. P., & Dohrenwend, B. S. *Social status and psychological disorder: A causal inquiry.* New York, Wiley, 1969.

23. Dohrenwend, B. P., Dohrenwend, B. S., Gould, M. S., Link, B., Neugebauer, R., & Wunsch-Hitzig, R. *Mental illness in the United States–Epidemiological estimates.* New York, Praeger, 1980.

24. Roth, W. F., & Luton, F. B. The mental hygiene program in Tennessee. *American Journal of Psychiatry*, **99**, 662–75 (1943).

25. Bremer, J. A. A social psychiatric investigation of a small community in northern

Norway. *Acta Psychiatrica et Neurologica Scandinavica Supplementum* 62 (1951).

26. Fremming, K. M. *The expectation of mental infirmity in a sample of the Danish population.* London, Eugenics Society, 1951.

27. Essen-Möller, E. Individual traits and morbidity in a Swedish rural population. *Acta Psychiatrica et Neurologica Scandinavica*, Suppl. 100 (1955).

28. Trussell, R. E., Elinson, J., & Levin, M. L. Comparisons of various methods of estimating the prevalence of chronic disease in a community; the Hunterdon County study. *American Journal of Public Health*, **46**, 173–82 (1956).

29. Pasamanick, B., Roberts, D. W., Lemkau, P. W., & Krueger, D. B. A survey of mental disease in an urban population: Prevalence by race and income. In B. Pasamanick (Ed.), *Epidemiology of mental disorder*. Washington, DC, American Association for the Advancement of Science, 1959. Pp. 183–91.

30. Llewellyn-Thomas, E. The prevalence of psychiatric symptoms within an island fishing village. *Canadian Medical Association Journal*, **93**, 197–204 (1960).

31. Primrose, A. J. R. *Psychological illness: A community study*. London, Tavistock, 1962.

32. Helgason, L. Psychiatric services and mental illness in Iceland. *Acta Psychiatrica Scandinavica*, Suppl. 268 (1977).

33. Hagnell, O. *A prospective study of the incidence of mental disorder*. Stockholm, Nordstedt, 1966.

34. Andersen, T. Physical and mental illness in a Lapp and Norwegian population. *Acta Psychiatrica Scandinavica*, Suppl. 263, pp. 47–56 (1975).

35. Fugelli, A. R. Mental health and living conditions in a fishing community in northern Norway. *Acta Psychiatrica Scandinavica*, Suppl. 263, pp. 39–42 (1975).

36. Edgerton, J. W., Bentz, W., & Hollister, W. Demographic factors and responses to stress among rural people. *American Journal of Public Health*, **60**, 1065–71 (1970).

37. Schwab, J. J., McGinnis, N. H., & Warheit, G. J. Social psychiatric impairment: Racial comparisons. *American Journal of Psychiatry*, **130**, 183–87 (1973).

38. Shore, J. H., Kinzie, J. D., Hampson, J. L., & Pattison, E. M. Psychiatric epidemiology of an Indian village. *Psychiatry*, **36**, 70–81 (1973).

39. Schwab, J. J., Bell, R. A., Warheit, G. J., & Schwab, R. B. *Social order and mental health*. New York, Brunner/Mazel, 1979.

40. Srole, L., Langner, T. S., Michael, S. T., Opler, M. K., & Rennie, T. A. C. *Mental health in the metropolis: The Midtown Manhattan study*. Vol. 1. New York, McGraw-Hill, 1962.

41. Phillips, D. L. The true prevalence of mental illness in a New England state. *Community Mental Health Journal,* **2**, 35–40 (1966).

42. Haese, P. N., & Meile, R. L. The relative effectiveness of two models for scoring the Midtown Psychological Index. *Community Mental Health Journal*, **3**, 335–42 (1967).

43. Meile, R. L., & Haese, P. N. Social status, status incongruence and symptoms of stress. *Journal of Health and Social Behaviour*, **10**, 237–44 (1969).

44. Phillips, D. L., & Segal, B. E. Social status and psychiatric illness. *American Sociological Review*, **34**, 58–72 (1969).

45. Summers, G. F., Seiler, L. H., & Hough, R. L. Psychiatric symptoms: Cross validation with a rural sample. *Rural Sociology*, **36**, 367–78 (1971).

46. Gaitz, C. M., & Scott, J. Age and the measurement of mental health. *Journal of Health and Social Behavior*, **13**, 55–67 (1972).

47. Yancey, W. L., Rigsby, L., & McCarthy, J. D. Social position and self-evaluation: The relative importance of race. *American Journal of Sociology*, **78**, 338–59 (1972).

48. Cole, N. J., Branch, C. H. H., & Orla, M. Mental illness. A survey assessment of community rates, attitudes and adjustments. *AMA Archives of Neurology and Psychiatry*, **77**, 393–98 (1957).

49. Brunetti, P. M. A prevalence survey of mental disorders in a rural commune in Vaucluse: Methodological considerations. *Acta Psychiatrica Scandinavica*, **40**, 323–58 (1964).

50. Taylor, L. H., & Chave, S. *Mental health and environment*. London, Longmans Green, 1964.

51. Hare, E. H., & Shaw, G. K. *Mental health on a new housing estate*. New York, Oxford University Press, 1965.

52. Piotrowski, A., Henisz, J., & Gnat, T. Individual interview and clinical examination to determine prevalence of mental disorders. Proceedings of the Fourth World Congress of Psychiatry, Madrid, 5–11 September 1966. *Excerpta Medica*, International Congress Series No. 150, pp. 2477–78.

53. Giel, R., & Le Nobel, C. P. J. Neurotic instability in a Dutch village. *Acta Psychiatrica Scandinavica*, **47**, 462–72 (1971).

54. Schwab, J. J., & Warheit, G. J. Evaluating southern mental health needs and services. *Journal of Florida Medical Association*, **59**, 17–20 (1972).

55. Bjarner, E., Rappesgaard, H., & Astrup, C. Psychiatric morbidity in Berlevag. *Acta Psychiatrica Scandinavica*, Suppl. 263, pp. 60–67 (1975).

56. Väisänen, E. Psychiatric disorders in Finland. *Acta Psychiatrica Scandinavica*, suppl. 263, pp. 22–23 (1975).

57. Schepank, H. Epidemiologie psychogener Erkrankungen. *Psychosomatische Medizin und Psychoanalyse*, **28**, 104–125 (1982).

58. Dohrenwend, B. P., Egri, G., & Mendelsohn, F. S. Psychiatric disorder in general populations: A study of the problem of clinical judgment. *American Journal of Psychiatry*, **127**, 1304–1312 (1971).

59. Weissman, M. M., Myers, J. K., & Harding, P. S. Psychiatric disorders in a United States urban community. *American Journal of Psychiatry*, **135**, 459–62 (1978).

60. Wing, J. K., Mann, S. A., Leff, J. P., & Nixon, J. M. The concept of a 'case' in psychiatric population surveys. *Psychological Medicine*, **8**, 203–217 (1978).

61. Finlay-Jones, R. A., & Burvill, P. W. The prevalence of minor psychiatric morbidity in the community. *Psychological Medicine*, **7**, 475–89 (1977).

62. Shiraer, N., & Armstrong, J. *Health care survey of Gosfordwyong and Illawarra 1975*. Sydney, Division of Health Services Research, Health Commission of New South Wales, 1978.

63. Henderson, A. S., Duncan-Jones, P., Byrne, D. G., & Scott, R. Measuring social relationships. The interviewer schedule for social interaction. *Psychological Medicine*, **10**, 723–34 (1980).

64. Leaf, P. J., Weissmann, M. M., Myers, I. K., Tischler, G. L., & Holzer, Ch. E. Social factors related to psychiatric disorder: The Yale Epidemiological Catchment Area Project. *Social Psychiatry*, **19**, 53–62 (1984).

65. American Psychiatric Association. *Diagnostic and statistical manual of mental disorders* (3rd ed.) (DSM-III). Washington, DC, American Psychiatric Association, 1980.

66. Cooper, B. Mental illness, disability and social conditions among old people in Mannheim. In H. Häfner, G. Moschel, & N. Sartorius (Eds.), *Mental health in the elderly. A review of the present state of research*. Berlin, Springer, 1986.

67. Henderson, A. S. Epidemiology of mental illness. In H. Häfner, G. Moschel, & N. Sartorius (Eds.), *Mental health in the elderly. A review of the present state of research*. Berlin, Springer, 1986.

68. Cooper, B., & Sosna, U. Psychische Erkrankungen in der Altenbevölkerung. Eine epidemiologische Feldstudie in Mannheim. *Nervenarzt*, **54**, 239–49 (1983).

69. Sheldon, J. H. *The social medicine of old age. Report of an inquiry in Wolverhampton*. London, Oxford University Press, 1948.

70. Nielsen, J. Gerontopsychiatric period-prevalence investigation in a geographically delimited population. *Acta Psychiatrica Scandinavica*, **38**, 307–330 (1962).

71. Kay, D. W. K., Beamish, P., & Roth, M. Old age mental disorders in Newcastle upon Tyne, Part I: A study of prevalence; Part II: A study of possible social and medical causes. *British Journal of Psychiatry*, **110**, 146–58 (1964).

72. Parsons, P. L. Mental health of Swansea's old folk. *British Journal of Preventive and Social Medicine*, **19**, 43–47 (1965).

73. Dilling, H., & Weyerer, S. *Behandelte und nicht behandelte psychiatrische Morbidität in der Bevölkerung. Bericht an die Deutsche Forschungsgemeinschaft über das Projekt A10*. Munich, Psychiatrische Klinik der Universität München, 1980.

74. Häfner, H. *Psychische Gesundheit im Alter*. Stuttgart, Gustav Fischer Verlag, 1986.

75. Kay, D. W. K., Bergmann, K., Foster, E. M., McKechnie, A. A., & Roth, M. Mental illness and hospital usage in the elderly: A random sample followed up. *Comprehensive Psychiatry*, **11**, 26–35 (1970).

76. Kaneko, Z. Care in Japan. In J. G. Howells (Ed.), *Modern perspectives in psychiatry of old age*. New York, Brunner/Mazel, 1975. Pp. 519–30.

77. New York State Department of Mental Hygiene. *A mental health survey of older people*. Utica, NY, State Hospitals Press, 1961.

78. Bickel, H., & Cooper, B. Psychische Erkrankung und Mortalität in der Altenbevölkerung. Vorläufige Ergebnisse einer Längsschnittstudie. 12. Tagung der europäischen Arbeitsgemeinschaft für Gerontopsychiatrie, Kassel, 5–8 September 1984. In H. Radebold (Ed.), *Janssen Symposion Gerontopsychiatrie*. Neuss, Janssen, 1986. Pp. 313–34.

79. Eastwood, M. R., & Trevelyan, M. H. Relationship between psychical and psychiatric disorder. *Psychological Medicine*, **2**, 363–72 (1972).

80. Andrews, G., Schonell, M., & Tennant, C. The relation between psychological and social morbidity in a suburban community. *American Journal of Epidemiology*, **105**, 324–29 (1977).

81. Cooper, B., Glettler, G., & Abt, H. G. Psychiatric disorder, physical impairments and disability among the elderly in an urban community. In G. Magnussen & J. Nielsen (Eds.), *Epidemiology and prevention of mental disorder in old age*. Hellerup, Denmark, EGV, 1982. Pp. 52–62.

82. Cooper, B., & Schwarz, R. Psychiatric case-identification in an elderly urban population. *Social Psychiatry*, **17**, 43–52 (1982).

83. Lansbury, I. The prevalence of physical disease in a large mental hospital and its implications for staffing. *Hospital & Community Psychiatry*, **23**, 148–51 (1972).

84. Maguire, G. P., & Granville-Grossman, U. L. Physical illness in psychiatric patients. *British Journal of Psychiatry*, **115**, 1365–69 (1968).

85. Munoz, R. A. Mental, medical and social problems in a psychiatric population. *Psychosomatics*, **17**, 194–96 (1976).

86. Kampmeier, R. H. Diagnosis and treatment of physical disease in the mentally ill. *Annals of Internal Medicine*, **86**, 637–45 (1977).

87. Lipowski, Z. J. Physical illness and psychiatric disorder: A neglected relationship. In K. Achte & A. Pakaslahti (Eds.), *Psychological factors in disease. Psychiatria Fennica*, Supplement (1979).

88. Shewitz, S. A., Silberfarb, P. M., & Lipowski, Z. J. Psychiatric consultations in a general hospital: A report of 1000 referrals. *Diseases of the Nervous System*, **37**, 295–300 (1976).

89. Kigerman, M. J., & McKegney, F. P. Patterns of psychiatric consultations in two general hospitals. *Psychiatric Medicine*, **2**, 126–32 (1971).

90. Tuason, V. B., & Rhee, Y. W. Psychiatric disorders in patients of a general hospital. *Southern Medical Journal*, **65**, 408–412 (1972).

91. Dovenmuehle, R. H., & Verwoerdt, A. Physical illness and depressive symptomatology. Incidence of depressive symptoms in hospitalized cardiac patients. *Journal of the American Geriatrics Society*, **10**, 932–47 (1962).

92. Sosna, U. *Soziale Isolation und psychische Erkrankungen im Alter. Eine medizinsoziologische Feldstudie in Mannheim*. Frankfurt, Campus Verlag, 1983.

93. Svanborg, A., Berg, S., Mellstöm, D., Nilsson, L., & Persson, G. Possibilities of preserving physical and mental fitness and autonomy in old age. In H. Häfner, G. Moschel, & N. Sartorius (Eds.), *Mental health in the elderly. A review of the present state of research*. Berlin, Springer, 1986.

94. Murphy, H. P. M. *Comparative psychiatry. The international and intercultural distribution of mental illness*. Berlin, Springer, 1982.

95. World Health Organization. *The international pilot study of schizophrenia*. Vol. 1. Geneva, World Health Organization, 1973.

96. World Health Organization. *Schizophrenia. An international follow-up study*. Chichester, Wiley & Simons, 1979.

97. Jablensky, A., Schwarz, R., & Tomov, J. WHO-collaborative study on impairments and disabilities associated with schizophrenic disorders. *Acta Psychiatrica Scandinavica*, Suppl. 285, pp. 152–63 (1980).

98. Jablensky, A., Multicultural studies and the nature of schizophrenia: a review. *Journal of the Royal Society of Medicine*, **80**, 162–167 (1987).

99.   Häfner, H., Welz, R., Gorenc, K., & Kleff, F. Selbstmordversuche und depressive Störungen. *Schweizer Archiv für Neurologie, Neurochirurgie und Psychiatrie,* **133,** 283–94 (1983).

100. Durkheim, E. *Suicide.* New York, The Free Press of Glencoe, 1951.

101. Pittman, B. J. International overview: Social and cultural factors in drinking patterns. In B. J. Pittman (Ed.), *Alcoholism.* New York, Harper & Row, 1967.

102. Bruun, K., Edwards, G., & Lumio, M. Alcohol control policies in public health perspective. *The Finnish Foundation for Alcohol Studies,* **25** (1975).

103. Nielsen, J., & Sorensen, K. Alcohol policy. Alcohol consumption, alcohol prices, delirium tremens and alcoholism as cause of death in Denmark. *Social Psychiatry,* **14,** 133–38 (1979).

104. Osuntokun, B. O. The value of collaborative research in aging. In H. Häfner, G. Moschel, & N. Sartorius (Eds.), *Mental health in the elderly: A review of the present state of research.* Berlin, Heidelberg, New York, Tokyo, Springer, 1986.

105. Wolin, S. J., Benett, L. A., Nooland, D. L., & Teitelbaum, M. S. Disrupted family rituals. *Journal of Studies on Alcohol,* **41,** 199–214 (1980).

106. Soer, J. von. *Jugendalkoholismus.* Weinheim, Beltz, 1980.

107. Smart, R. G., & Fejer, D. Drug use among adolescents and their parents. Closing the generation gap in mood modification. *Journal of Abnormal Psychology,* **79,** 153–60 (1972).

108. Kandel, D. Interpersonal influences on adolescent illegal drug use. In E. Josephson & E. Carroll (Eds.), *Drug use: Epidemiological and sociological approaches.* Washington, DC, Hemisphere, 1974. Pp. 207–240.

109. Gorsuch, R. L. Interactive models of nonmedical drug use. In D. J. Lettieri, M. Sayers, & H. Pearson Wallenstein (Eds.), *Theories on drug abuse.* Rockville, MD, National Institute on Drug Abuse, 1980. Pp. 18–23.

110. Andrews, K. H., & Kandel, D. B. Attitude and behavior: A specification of the contingent consistency theory. *American Sociological Review,* **44,** 298–310 (1979).

111. Alarcon, de R. The spread of heroin in a community. *Bulletin on Narcotics.* **21,** 17–22 (1969).

112. Levengood, R., Lowinger, P., & Schooff, K. Heroin addiction in the suburbs – An epidemiological study. *American Journal of Public Health,* **36,** 209–214 (1973).

113. Hughes, P. H., Crawford, G. A., & Jaffe, J. H. Heroin epidemics in Chicago. In *Proceedings of the World Congress of Psychiatry, Mexico City. Excerpta Medica,* 1416–24 (1971).

114. Hughes, P. H., & Crawford, G. A. A contagious disease model of researching and intervening in heroin epidemics. *Archives of General Psychiatry,* **27,** 149–55 (1972).

115. Welz, R. *Drogen, Alkohol und Suizid.* Stuttgart, Enke, 1983.

116. Chambers, C. D., & Hunt, L. G. *The heroin epidemics.* New York, Spectrum, 1976.

117. Rogers, E. M., & Schoemaker, F. F. *Communications of innovations. A cross cultural approach.* New York, McGraw-Hill, 1971.

118. Faris, R. E. L., & Dunham, W. H. *Mental disorders in urban areas.* Chicago, University of Chicago Press, 1939.

119. Chein, I., Gerard, D. L., Lee, R. S. & Rosenfeld, E. *The road to heroin.* New York, Essex Books, 1964.

120. Richman, A. Ecological studies on narcotic addiction. In L. G. Richards & L. B. Blevens (Eds.), *The epidemiology of drug abuse.* Research Monographs, No. 10. Rockville, MD, National Institute on Drug Abuse, 1977. Pp. 173–96.

121. Cavan, R. S. *Suicide.* Chicago, University of Chicago Press, 1928.

122. Sainsbury, P. *Suicide in London.* London, Chapman & Hall, 1955.

123. McCarthy, P. D., & Walsh, D. Suicide in Dublin. *Journal of the Irish Medical Association,* **57**, 8–13 (1965).

124. Lester, D. Social disorganization and completed suicide. *Social Psychiatry,* **5**, 175–76 (1970).

125. Buglass, D., & Duffy, J. C. The ecological pattern of suicide and parasuicide in Edinburgh. *Social Science & Medicine.* **12**, 241–53 (1978).

126. Welz, R. Suicidal areas: cluster analysis profiles of urban environments. *Acta Psychiatrica Scandinavica,* Suppl. 285, pp. 372–81 (1980).

127. Brugger, C. Versuch einer Geisteskrankenzählung in Thüringen. *Zeitschrift für die gesamte Neurologie und Psychiatrie,* **133**, 352–90 (1931).

128. Brugger, C. Psychiatrische Bestandsaufnahme im Gebiet eines medizinisch-anthropologischen Zensus in der Nähe von Rosenheim. *Zeitschrift für die gesamte Neurologie und Psychiatrie,* **160**, 189–207 (1938).

129. Tietze, C., Lemkau, P. V., & Cooper, M. Schizophrenia, manic depressive psychoses and social economic status. *American Journal of Sociology,* **47**, 167–74 (1941).

130. Hollingshead, A., & Redlich, F. C. *Social class and mental illness.* New York, Wiley, 1958.

131. Schroeder, C. W. Mental disorders in cities. *American Journal of Sociology,* **48**, 40–42 (1942).

132. Gardner, E. A., & Babigian, H. M. A longitudinal comparison of psychiatric service. *American Journal of Orthopsychiatry,* **36**, 818 (1966).

133. Dunham, H. W. *Community and schizophrenia: An epidemiological analysis.* Detroit, MI, Wayne State University Press, 1965.

134. Sundby, P., & Nyhus, P. Major and minor psychiatric disorders in males in Oslo. *Acta Psychiatrica Scandinavica,* **39**, 519–47 (1963).

135. Walsh, D., & Walsh, B. Mental illness in the Republic of Ireland: First admissions. *Journal of the Irish Medical Association,* **63**, 365–70 (1970).

136. Häfner, H., & Reimann, H. Spatial distribution of mental disorders in Mannheim, 1965. In E. H. Hare & J. K. Wing (Eds.), *Psychiatric epidemiology* (Proceedings of an international symposium held at Aberdeen University, July 1969). London, Oxford University Press, 1970. Pp. 341–54.

137. Cooper, B., & Lackus, B. The social-class background of mentally retarded children. A study in Mannheim. *Social Psychiatry,* **19**, 3–12 (1984).

138. Odegard, O. Social and ecological factors in the etiology, outcome, treatment

and prevention of mental disorders. In K. P. Kisker, J. E. Meyer, C. Müller, & E. Strömgren (Eds.), *Psychiatrie der Gegenwart.* Berlin, Heidelberg, New York, Springer, 1975. Vol. III, pp. 151–98.

139. Dai, B. *Opium addiction in Chicago.* Montclair, NJ, Patterson Smith, 1970 (first published in 1937).

140. Dietrich, H., & Herle, L. Über Alter, Sozialschicht, Mobilität und Wohnort chronischer Alkoholiker. *Kölner Zeitschrift für Soziologie und Sozialpsychologie,* **15**, 277–94 (1963).

141. Langner, T. S., & Michael, S. T. *Life stress and mental health. The Midtown Manhattan Study.* Glencoe, IL, The Free Press, 1963.

142. Welz, R. *Selbstmorbversuche in städtischen Lebensumwelten.* Weinheim, Beltz, 1979.

143. Clausen, J. A., & Kohn, M. L. Relation of schizophrenia to the social structure of a small city. In B. Pasamanick (Ed.), *Epidemiology of mental disorder.* Washington, DC, American Association for the Advancement of Science, 1959.

144. Goldberg, E. M., & Morrison, S. L. Schizophrenia and social class. *British Journal of Psychiatry,* **109**, 765–802 (1963).

145. Turner, R., & Wagenfeld, M. O. Occupational mobility and schizophrenia: An assessment of the social causation and selection hypotheses. *American Sociological Review,* **32**, 114 (1967).

146. Häfner, H. Der Einfluss von Umweltfaktoren auf das Erkrankungsrisiko für Schizophrenie. *Nervenarzt,* **42**, 557–68 (1971).

147. Häfner, H., & an der Heiden, W. The contribution of European case registers to research on schizophrenia. *Schizophrenia Bulletin,* **12**, 26–51 (1986).

148. Goodman, A. B., Siegel, M. S. C., Graig, T. J., & Lin, S. P. The relationship between socioeconomic class and prevalence of schizophrenia, alcoholism, and affective disorders treated by inpatient care in a suburban area. *American Journal of Psychiatry* **140**, 166–70 (1983).

149. Dalgard, O. S. *Migration and functional psychoses in Oslo.* Oslo, Universitetsforlaget, 1971.

150. Lane, E. A. & Albee, G. W. Childhood intellectual differences between schizophrenic adults and their siblings. *American Journal of Orthopsychiatry,* **35**, 747 (1965).

151. Kringlen, E. *Heredity and environment in the functional psychoses.* Oslo, Universitetsforlaget, 1969.

152. Slater, E. *Psychotic and neurotic illness in twins* (Medical Research Council, Special Report Series No. 278). London, HMSO, 1953.

153. Kringlen, E. Schizophrenia in male monozygotic twins. *Acta Psychiatrica Scandinavica Supplementum* 178 (1964).

154. Tienari, P. Psychiatric illness in identical twins. *Acta Psychiatrica Scandinavica Supplementum* 171 (1963).

155. Tienari, P. Schizophrenia in Finnish male twins. In M. H. Lader (Ed.), *Studies of schizophrenia. British Journal of Psychiatry,* Special Publication No. 10. Kent, Asford, Headley Brothers, 1975. Pp. 29–35.

156. Rosenthal, D., Wender, P., Kety, S. S., Schulsinger, F., Welner, J., & Ostergard, L. Schizophrenics' offspring reared in adoptive homes. In D. Rosenthal & S. S. Kety (Eds.), *The transmission of schizophrenia*. Oxford, Pergamon Press, 1968. Pp. 377–91.

157. Fischer, M., Harvald, B., & Hauge, M. A Danish twin study of schizophrenia. *British Journal of Psychiatry*, **115**, 981–90 (1969).

158. Mechanic, D. *Medical sociology. A selective view*. New York, The Free Press, 1968.

159. McKinlay, J. B. Social networks, lay consultations and help-seeking behaviour. *Social Forces*, **51**, 275–92 (1973).

160. Suchman, E. Social patterns and medical care. *Journal of Human Behavior*, **6**, 2–16 (1965).

161. Reimann, H., & Häfner, H. Psychische Erkrankungen alter Menschen in Mannheim. *Social Psychiatry*, **7**, 53–69 (1972).

162. Moeller, M. L. *Selbsthilfegruppen. Selbstbehandlung und Selbsterkenntnis in eigenverantwortlichen Kleingruppen*. Reinbeck, Rowohlt, 1978.

163. Siegrist, J. Die Bedeutung von Lebensereignissen für die Entstehung körperlicher und psychosomatischer Erkrankungen. *Nervenarzt*, **51**, 313–20 (1980).

164. Paykel, E. S., Prusoff, B. A., & Myers, J. K. Suicide attempts and recent life events. *Archives of General Psychiatry*, **32**, 327–33 (1975).

165. Kuhnt, S., Kleff, F., & Welz, R. Stressbelastung und Stressbewältigungsressourcen bei Individuen mit suizidalen Handlungen. In G. Luer (Ed.), *Bericht über den 33. Kongress der Deutschen Gesellschaft für Psychologie*. Göttingen, Hogrefe, 1983.

166. Jahoda, M., Lazarsfeld, P. S., & Zeisel, H. *Die Arbeitslosen von Marienthal*. Allensbach, Bonn, Verlag für Demoskopie, 1960.

167. Cobb, S., & Gore, S. *Unemployment, social support and health*. Ann Arbor, MI, University of Michigan, Survey Research Center, 1973.

168. Cobb, S. Social support as a moderator of life stress. *Psychosomatic Medicine*, **38**, 300–314 (1976).

169. Gore, S. The effect of social support in moderating the health consequences of unemployment. *Journal of Health and Social Behavior*, **19**, 157–65 (1978).

170. Pearlin, L. J., & Schooler, C. The structure of coping. *Journal of Health and Social Behavior*, **19**, 2–21 (1978).

171. Astrup, C., & Odegard, O. Internal migration and mental disease in Norway. *Psychiatric Quarterly*, suppl. 34, pp. 116–30 (1960).

172. Eitinger, L., & Grünfeld, B. Psychoses among refugees in Norway. *Acta Psychiatrica Scandinavica*, **42**, 315–28 (1966).

173. Häfner, H., Moschel, G., & Özek, M. Psychische Störungen bei türkischen Gastarbeitern. Eine retrospektiv-epidemiologische Studie zur Untersuchung der Reaktion auf Einwanderung und partielle Anpassung. *Nervenarzt*, **48**, 268–75 (1977).

174. Pflanz, M., Hasenkopf, O., & Costas, P. Blutdruck und funktionelle Beschwerden bei Gastarbeitern – Ein transkultureller Vergleich. *Arbeitsmedizin Sozialmedizin Arbeitshygiene*, **5**, 181–85 (1967).

175. Binder, J., & Simoes, M. Sozialpsychiatrie der Gastarbeiter. *Fortschritte der Neurologie-Psychiatrie*, **46**, 342–59 (1978).

176. Häfner, H. Psychiatrische Morbidität von Gastarbeitern. *Nervenarzt*, **51**, 672–83 (1980).

177. Häfner, H. Are mental disorders increasing over time? *Psychopathology*, **18**, 66–81 (1985).

178. Goldhamer, H., & Marshall, A. *Psychoses and civilization.* Glencoe, IL, The Free Press, 1953.

179. Dunham, H. W. Society, culture and mental disorder. *Archives of General Psychiatry*, **32**, 147–56 (1976).

180. Kramer, M., von Korff, M., & Kessler, L. G. The lifetime prevalence of mental disorders: Estimation, uses and limitations, *Psychiatry in Medicine*, **10**, 429–35 (1980).

181. Torrey, E. F. *Schizophrenia and civilization.* New York and London, J. Aronson, 1980.

182. Eaton, W. W. *The sociology of mental disorders.* New York, Praeger, 1980.

183. Krupinski, J., & Alexander, L. Patterns of psychiatric morbidity in Victoria, Australia, in relation to changes in diagnostic criteria 1948–1978. *Social Psychiatry*, **18**, 61–67 (1983).

184. Klug, J. *Psychiatrische Diagnosen,* Weinheim, Beltz, 1983.

185. Helgason, T. Psychiatric services and mental illness in Iceland. *Acta Psychiatrica Scandinavica*, Suppl. 1 (2) **268**, 1977.

186. Wing, J. K. & Fryers, T. (Eds). *Psychiatric services in Camberwell and Salford. Statistics from the Camberwell and Salford psychiatric registers, 1964–1974.* London, MRC Social Psychiatry Unit and Department of Community Medicine, University of Manchester (1976).

187. Munk-Jörgensen, P. Schizophrenia in Denmark. Incidence and utilization of psychiatric institutions, *Acta Psychiatrica Scandinavica* **73**, 172–180. (1986).

188. Giel, R., Sauer, H. C., Slooff, C. J., & Wiersma, D. Epidemiological observations on schizophrenia and disability in the Netherlands. *Tijdschrift voor Psychiatrie*, **11–12**, 710–22 (1980).

189. Tansella, M., Faccincani, C., Mignolli, G., Balestrieri, M., & Zimmermann-Tansella, C. Il registro psichiatrico di Verona-Sud. Epidemiologia per la valutazione dei nuovi servizi territoriali. In M. Tansella (Ed.), *L'Approccio epidemiologico in psichiatria.* Torino, Boringhieri, 1985. Pp. 225–59.

190. Warthen, F. J., Klee, G. D., Bahn, A. K., & Gorwitz, K. *Diagnosed schizophrenia in Maryland* (Psychiatric Research Report 22). Washington, DC, American Psychiatric Association, 1967.

191. Babigian, H. M. Schizophrenia: Epidemiology. In A. M. Freedman, H. I. Kaplan, & B. J. Sadock (Eds.), *Comprehensive textbook of psychiatry*, II. Baltimore, Williams & Wilkins, 1975. Pp. 860–66.

192. Dilling, H., Weyerer, S. & Lissio, H. Zur ambulanten psychiatrischen Versorgung durch niedergelassene Nervenärzte. *Social Psychiatry* **10**, 111–131 (1975).

193. Eaton, W. Epidemiology of schizophrenia. *Epidemiologic Reviews* **7**, 105–126 (1985).

2

Food-related behaviour

M. Abdussalam, C. Foster & F. Käferstein

Food is one of the most important determinants of health, and people everywhere hold beliefs about this relationship. They endeavour to select, prepare, and consume food in ways they believe to be consistent with health promotion and protection. Unfortunately, however, many food beliefs and practices are not in accord with scientific concepts of balanced nutrition and hygiene (safety). Although the types, varieties, and quantities of food available to a community are determined largely by ecological, economic (including trade), and technological factors, food habits and beliefs – i.e. food-related behaviour – strongly influence what is actually consumed, and in what forms and quantities. These habits and beliefs therefore have major implications for health-promoting aspects of food and for the prevention of malnutrition and food-borne diseases.

Food habits formed under particular social and economic conditions, and entirely adequate to those conditions, may be carried by individuals and groups into other settings where they may be unsuitable and even harmful to health. For example, rural or tribal people moving to towns, or migrant workers, tourists, or refugees living for varying periods in strange communities, may face health problems because of their food habits or may cause difficulties for the host communities. Although food habits change constantly under various pressures, it is well to realize that dietary beliefs are among the most resistant to change, and that it is often extremely difficult to hasten changes in food habits, even when those habits constitute serious health hazards. It is therefore necessary for health workers to understand the basic factors involved in the formation and modification of food habits and the principles on which interventions for inducing changes can be based and carried out.

Dr Abdussalam is a former staff member of the World Health Organization, now retired; Dr Foster is Professor Emeritus, Department of Anthropology, University of California, Berkeley, California; and Dr Käferstein is Manager, Food Safety Unit, Division of Environmental Health, World Health Organization, Geneva, Switzerland.

Determinants of food-related behaviour

Human behaviour as it relates to food embraces a complex of culinary activities and patterns of consumption resulting from the interaction of ecological, economic, technological, and social factors. The most important determinants can be divided into two groups: factors stemming from the sociocultural context, and factors stemming from the individual (physiological or psychological) context.

The sociocultural role of food

The primary function of food is to sustain life. Yet, in every society, dietary customs play basic social and symbolic roles that far transcend mere nourishment of the human body. Therefore, in searching for solutions to the world's nutritional and associated food safety problems, food-related behaviour must be viewed as a biosocial phenomenon involving both the biological and the behavioural sciences.

In this section we are concerned primarily with the latter, the behavioural components of human food activities. Specifically, we shall deal with (a) the cultural definition and classification of foods, (b) traditional beliefs and practices as they affect nutrition and health, and (c) the symbolic roles of food that contribute to the integration of social and political units – of nations, communities, and families.

Definition and classification of food

'Food' is a cultural concept; 'nutrient', a biological one. The natural environments of all human groups provide a variety of nutrients, or the potential to produce them. But nutrients do not become food until they are so defined by culture, that is, are certified as fit for human consumption. No group, perhaps not even under conditions of extreme starvation, utilizes every available nutritional substance (see, for example, Jelliffe & Bennett (1) on the Hadza hunters of Tanzania). Because of historical reasons, religious taboos, health beliefs, and the like, at least some nutritionally valuable items are excluded from every customary diet.

To illustrate: In the United States, perhaps because of the country's multi-ethnic origins and an abundantly productive food system, an astonishingly wide variety of nutrients have been classified as 'food', and are available for the daily table. Yet many nutritious items, highly esteemed by members of other societies, are not defined as food by most Americans. Among those that come to mind are horse meat, dogs, dolphins, sheep eyes, armadillos, salamanders, rattlesnakes, iguanas, small birds such as larks and warblers, mare's and ewe's milk, sea urchins, eels, seaweed, ants and grubs, cassava (except as tapioca), millet, quinoa, and amaranth. As an academic exercise, and drawing upon the world's resources, an adequate human diet could be formulated from foods rarely, if ever, eaten by the average American.

Foods are not just culturally defined: they are also classified. Classification is essential because it specifies how, where, when, and by whom, each food or type of food can be eaten, thus providing the rationale for the prescriptions and proscriptions that characterize every dietary system. By means of culturally determined classifications, the members of every society know the appropriate foods for each meal of the day, for between-meal snacks, and for ritual feasting. They also know the prescribed and proscribed foods at times of illness, during pregnancy and the post-partum period, and for the several stages of the life cycle.

The characteristics of food that determine whether it is appropriate or inappropriate for specific events and conditions include inherent qualities thought to reside in the food itself, such as 'lightness' versus 'heaviness', and 'nutritious' versus 'non-nutritious'. One of the most widespread and complex of all food classificatory systems describes foods as either 'heating' or 'cooling' according to the perceived effect on the human body. This system is found in traditional Chinese medicine, in Ayurveda and Unani medicine on the Indo-Pakistan subcontinent and in other parts of Southeast Asia, and in Latin American humoral pathology. At least two billion people are guided, to a greater or lesser extent, by this system in behaviour related to nutrition, growth, health, illness, pregnancy, and the post-partum period. Hot–cold rules present some of the knottiest problems in achieving balanced diets; many of the proscriptions, such as frequent reduction in protein intake during illness, are at odds with scientific conclusions on this subject. Yet humoral systems, because they are internally so consistent, provide logical frameworks for health education and other interventions designed to improve nutrition.

In most societies, at least some foods are classified according to a high-status versus low-status scale. Unfortunately, many high-status foods are often those that, through excessive milling and other forms of processing, have been deprived of much of their nutritional value. In other instances, highly nutritious foods such as quinoa have been rejected (e.g. in Bolivia) by the middle and upper classes, to whom they are readily available, because they are considered to be 'low class' (2). Similarly, Jelliffe (3) reports that poor people in West Bengal have rejected highly nutritious, inexpensive, pond fish they consider to be 'snakelike', and hence 'low class', in favour of expensive fish of no greater nutritional value.

Perceived status of food appears to have a more powerful effect on changing dietary patterns than do beliefs or knowledge about food's effect on health. This is important knowledge for those involved in nutrition education, for new or altered foods that can be invested with high status – through packaging, radio and television advertising, and health messages – are more apt to be adopted than neutral or low-status foods.

Traditional beliefs and practices

Where population pressures have not been excessive, and where environmental and climatic uncertainties are not extreme, traditional peoples have usually done a remarkably good job in developing adequate diets (4, 5). Through trial and error over generations they have acquired a folk wisdom that guides them in their definitions and classification of food, and in the ways food is prepared and consumed. Folk wisdom also often guides them in safe culinary practices, such as cooking meat in small pieces to effect maximum heat penetration, utilization of proper fermentation processes, thorough reheating of previously cooked foods for later consumption, and the like.

But folk wisdom is not an absolute guide to healthy food habits, and some widely held traditional ideas do not conform to what science considers the best dietary practices. Failure to recognize the *positive* relationship between nutritious, sanitary food and the health of its consumers is all too common. For example, we read that among the Adhola of Uganda, 'There is no conception of the differential nutritional value of foodstuffs. The Adhola see no link between nutrition ... and health .... There is no Adhola belief that illness can be caused by *lack* of a particular type of food' (6).

Most traditional peoples think in terms of quantity, of the feeling of a full stomach, not of quality. Thus, 'The people of Chinaura [pseudonym of a village in Lucknow District, India] generally believe that it is the adequate quantity of food that is important. The idea of quality is restricted to certain foods recognized to be "strengthening"' (7).

Often fruits and vegetables are believed to have little food value; they are eaten because they taste good, or are refreshing; but they are considered a luxury, not an essential item. And, as noted above, during times of illness many customary foods may be eliminated from the patient's diet. Often the items eliminated are those that the patient badly needs, especially protein and vitamins. In general, it appears that in most traditional societies there is little knowledge of deficiency conditions.

Failure to recognize the special nutritional needs of children has also been noted as a shortcoming in some traditional societies (8). Usually children are viewed as 'little adults', who stand in line for what is left over after father and other adults have eaten. Religious customs as well as folk belief may also handicap children, as in Bengal, where delays in the *mukhe bhat*, 'first rice', ceremony, which ought to occur at about the age of six months, prevents the addition of badly needed supplemental foods for the growing child (3).

Many customary kitchen practices and food preferences contribute to lack of safety in food preparation and eating. These include a predilection in some societies for raw fish and undercooked meats, the storage of perishable food at ambient temperatures, and the cook's failure to wash his or her hands before preparing food. Cultural beliefs as well as a shortage of water may contribute to this last problem. In much of Latin America, hands are thought to be heated by contact with pressing irons and pottery kilns or by working with metaphorically 'hot' substances such as mineral lime. Exposing 'hot' hands to cold water is believed to cause cramps and rheumatism, so people refrain from washing, often for many hours.

Symbolic roles of food

Food not only maintains life and promotes health but also has expressive functions, such as the reaffirmation of social ties, the sanctioning of religious beliefs and practices, and the expression of national and ethnic identities, which are essential to every society. Everywhere social ties are validated and maintained by the exchange of goods and services. Food is usually the favored gift: symbolically, to offer food is to offer love, affection, or friendship. To accept food so offered is to acknowledge the feelings expressed and to commit oneself to reciprocity. To withhold food or to fail to offer it in a context where it is expected is a symbolic expression of anger or hostility. Similarly, to reject proffered food may be interpreted as expressing hostile feelings toward the giver. People feel most secure when eating with friends and family, both in public and in private. Normally, we do not eat with our enemies.

Religious and ethnic affiliations are continually expressed through food customs. Hindu avoidance of beef, Moslem and Jewish taboos against pork, and the historic Catholic proscription of meat on Fridays and other feast days help identify individuals as members of religious groups. In the secular area, festive occasions are almost invariably marked by foods that are deemed especially appropriate for the occasion. In Mexico the insistence on turkey or chicken in *mole* sauce as the main course for wedding and baptismal feasts is an expression of the Mexican ethos, a symbolic recognition of Mexican cultural characteristics not shared by other societies. In the United States the annual Thanksgiving dinner must conform to a rather rigid model: 'turkey and all the trimmings'.

Most people feel that eating should be a happy, even joyous, occasion, often combining religious and social elements. It is not surprising that in the English language 'feast' and 'festival' derive from the same Latin root. Clearly, food-related behaviour cannot be fully comprehended without an awareness of the symbolic and social roles of foods and their modes of consumption.

Physiological and psychological factors

Physiological and psychological factors are more universal determinants of food-related behaviour than are the sociocultural elements, with which they frequently interact. It is well known that the appearance, smell, taste, temperature, and texture of foods play an important part in determining their acceptance, or the preference for some items rather than others. Sometimes sounds of frying or crackling cause a pleasant anticipatory sensation and draw attention to the food being prepared.

Taste and smell are closely associated, and are the principal physiological determinants of food preference. The taste buds, which react to different types of stimuli (salty, sour, sweet, and bitter), along with the olfactory epithelium, contribute to the perception of 'flavour' or palatability. Perhaps an important role of these senses is to help to distinguish spoiled, stale, or altered foods from wholesome ones; but they also lead to appreciation of delicacies and favourite foods.

The appearance of food is important and conditions the consumer to expect a certain type of palatability when the food is consumed, the expectation being based on previous experience. Packaging also has an important influence on the selection of food.

The texture of food, even in the absence of taste, can be a positive factor in determining preference. Water chestnuts, for example, are much appreciated in southern Asia not because of their marked taste, but because of their crispness. European equivalents may be the 'hardtack' of Scandinavia, or celery hearts elsewhere. A soft, butterlike texture is also much appreciated in most societies.

In many parts of the world, food causing mild pain stimuli, such as chili peppers and sharp curries or highly peppered dishes, are much appreciated, whereas those causing intense pain (acid foods, very sharp dishes) are considered unpleasant.

Consumers' taste also determines the amount of salt and sugar added to foods that have to be stored for some time; and these two common ingredients, along with water activity, affect the survival or multiplication of microorganisms in foods, with consequences for safety. In addition, they have important metabolic consequences.

Some *psychological* factors are derived from physiological determinants, but others are independent, or more psychological than physiological. Most people avoid new foods or accept them with hesitation; rejection of tinned food and even frozen food (other than ice cream) is frequently observed in rural areas of developing countries. During one of the famines in southern Asia, Western journalists reported that villagers refused the tinned fish the journalists offered them, though they were in a precarious, near-starvation condition.

Market studies have shown that apart from buying capacity, several psychological factors determine the choice of food by consumers. An important role is played by the appearance and presentation of food and the choice and quantity of the same item on display: large quantities suggest fresh supplies; small quantities give the impression of being left-overs. The buying list is determined mainly by the housewife and, to some extent, by the husband; children influence the list by refusing some items of food.

Most people prefer clean and wholesome food with flavours universally considered to be pleasant. Some communities, however, have developed a taste for strongly flavoured foods (cheeses, fermented fish, haggis, etc) that have been fermented to the point of being rotten. There are places where milk or milk products are stored in strong-smelling goat skins, food is spiced with asafoetida, or rancid butter is added to tea. Garlic is much appreciated in some societies but not in others.

As noted above, prestige is one of the most potent motives in food behaviour, especially when food is consumed in the presence of other members of the community or with their knowledge (9). Each culture has a prestige scale for different food items and for ways of consuming or presenting them. The European style of eating is still highly prestigious in the now-independent former colonies of European powers. Some low-caste Hindu groups may give up animal food and become vegetarians like high-caste Hindus when they climb up the social ladder (7). Examples of this phenomenon are readily found in both industrialized and developing societies.

Changing food habits
Patterns of food consumption and related behaviour of individuals and communities are constantly changing, though these changes are generally gradual and slow. This area of human behaviour is rather poorly studied, and a systematic history of human nutritional development is still to be written. Nevertheless, some recent changes in the food habits of various groups or communities can be noted, despite the fragmentary information currently available.

Such changes can be termed 'spontaneous', although they are induced by a wide variety of factors affecting individuals (age, health, economic and social status, culture, environment, migration, etc) or the community (agriculture, food gathering, technology and industry, emergencies, social and physical environment, etc). These factors are too numerous to be discussed in full here, so we shall deal only with some of the more important recent phenomena, such as urbanization, migrations, rapid economic and social changes, and progress in the technology of food production, processing, and distribution.

It is important to understand the nature of spontaneous changes in food habits and their underlying causes in order to be able to plan meaningful interventions for correcting behaviour that may be harmful to health. It has been observed that *induced* changes are likely to be successful only if they are not contrary to accepted social norms and, preferably, conform to the trends of spontaneous changes that have been taking place.

Urbanization
One of the most dramatic and important demographic phenomena of our time is the migration of people from rural and tribal areas to towns, and from smaller towns to big cities, some 800 of which have more than a million inhabitants –

many, more than five million. The phenomenon is especially marked in the developing world, where the urban population will have increased from 20% in 1950 to 43% by the year 2000 (10). The unfavourable public health and social consequences of this migration are manifested particularly in the overcrowded slums within cities and in the shanty towns on their outskirts. The demographic and socioeconomic characteristics of urban populations and of their physical environment have been discussed in several United Nations and World Bank publications (see Austin (10) for references) and by Velimirovic (11), who has also dealt with the hygienic and epidemiological aspects of urbanization.

The factors that determine the food behaviour of city-dwellers are numerous and complex, but most important is the consumer's socioeconomic level. Other significant factors are the community of origin of a migrant and the connections maintained with it (family), the human environment in the eating establishment (family, canteen, workplace, etc), length of stay in the city, and the educational–cultural level of the person.[1]

Well-to-do urban inhabitants consume a wide variety of foods, including abundant animal proteins and fresh fruits and vegetables. They increasingly use prepared and semiprepared foods, which are less subject to seasonal variations and may be more innovative than traditional products. In most countries this group tends to be concerned with reducing its calorie intake; but high-cholesterol, fatty, and refined foods are still common, and contribute to relatively high rates of obesity, diabetes, ischaemic heart disease, and other chronic conditions.

Less-privileged urban dwellers spend a major part of their income on food (up to 82% in a city in India, according to Thimmayama & co-workers (12)). They depend largely on the food available in the markets; even in peripheral shantytowns, they have little access to foods that rural populations can gather in nature. And, because the food in the markets may be beyond their limited resources, nutritional deficiencies among these people are very common.

The evidence regarding the incidence of malnutrition in urban compared with rural areas is inconclusive. Hendrickse (8), Jelliffe & Bennett (13), Jelliffe (3), and Richards (14), among others, believe that urbanization leads to dietary deterioration. In a more recent review, Austin (10) concludes that malnutrition is more common in rural than in urban areas in most countries, but that the incidence is accelerating more rapidly and the degree of deficiency is more severe among urban than rural people. In the face of widely divergent reports, it seems unwise to make generalizations on this complex topic. Whatever the prevalence in specific locations, children, pregnant and lactating women, and, often, older people are particularly affected.

A large part of the diet of the urban poor consists of staples such as cereals and tubers, supplemented by legumes or seafoods. Meat, eggs, poultry, dairy products, and other expensive commodities are consumed only rarely and on special occasions. Both because of limited financial resources and the common absence of storage facilities, food is purchased frequently and in small quantities from retail shops or from hawkers or street vendors. Consequently, the urban poor are more liable to face the problem of adulteration than are members of the wealthier sectors.

The high cost of fuel for cooking facilities in the homes of the urban poor sometimes leads to heating insufficient to kill pathogenic microorganisms or to destroy heat-labile toxins. Poor housing, non-availability of safe water, and unsatisfactory waste disposal, in the presence of vermin, insects, and environmental contaminants, increase the risk of food-borne disease, which is particularly harmful to children already suffering from malnutrition.

As previously mentioned, economic factors largely determine the choice of food, but other factors do influence the selection of items within the buyer's reach. Traditional beliefs and preferences play an important role, especially among recent arrivals to an area, who often pay higher prices for familiar items even when similar but unfamiliar and cheaper ones may be available.[2] Unfamiliar foods are more readily accepted in common kitchens, canteens, etc; but most families tend to stick to traditional foods, which they prepare at home.

In most developing societies, the head of the family and other adult bread-earners, usually males, have precedence in food selection and generally are served first at family meals. This tendency may weaken if the wife also works and earns money, but the children have lower priority in either case. Moreover, the working mother may leave the smaller children in the care of older ones during her absence, which may add to their unsatisfactory care and feeding.

Both among urban slum-dwellers and rural peoples, traditional beliefs about pregnant and lactating women often adversely affect these women's diet. During the latter part of pregnancy and, particularly, during the post-partum period, traditional diets tend to be heavily restricted. In societies in which foods are classified in a humoral sense as 'hot' or 'cold', new mothers are thought to be in a cold condition because of loss of blood and separation from the 'hot' foetus, now an infant. Often these mothers are denied 'cold' foods, which usually include the common fruits and vegetables (15). But 'very hot' foods, which include most sources of animal protein (16), are also sometimes denied mothers, because it is believed that they heat her milk and injure the nursing infant.

In many traditional societies breast feeding is generally continued for one to two years (or up to the second term of a subsequent pregnancy), and supplementary feeding does not generally start before six months. These long periods may have been adopted as a result of the prevalence of enteric infections, so dangerous for sucklings. In certain classes of poor city-dwellers, bottle feeding of infants is being adopted, in imitation of the more-affluent citizens, as a matter of prestige. Other dietary changes take place for the same reason.

International migrations

Migration across national borders is an old phenomenon, but it has assumed tremendous dimensions since World War 2. Recent migrants include three main categories: workers migrating to rich industrialized countries or to those with important mineral resources; tourists and other temporary visitors, such as pilgrims and congress participants; refugees from war-stricken or other disaster areas, mainly in Africa and Asia.

What follows essentially applies also to migrations *within* large countries.

Migrant workers

During the past two or three decades, millions of people have moved from developing countries to industrialized and other rich countries in search of work. In addition, an unknown (but considerable) number have moved from one developing country to another for varying lengths of time. In fact, migration across international borders is an extension of national migration from poorer to more prosperous areas. For this reason, the change in the behaviour of migrant workers is in many ways similar to that discussed under urbanization. There are, however, some aspects of the change that may be more prominent in international migration than in migration to towns within a country.

The migrant worker generally goes to live in another culture and has to abide by cultural and legal norms many of which are foreign to his home culture. Behaviour that is normal in the home setting may be considered abnormal (or at least peculiar) in the host country. With regard to food practices, the migrant often has to adapt to new methods of cooking and food processing, use new types of food commodities, and learn to appreciate new and often strange dishes that differ in appearance and taste from those to which he is accustomed, especially if he has to eat outside the home in common kitchens, canteens, etc. Migrants living in families can prepare dishes to their own taste, but often have to use local ingredients. The transition is less abrupt in places where large colonies of compatriot migrants have already settled, e.g. in Chinatowns, German, Italian, or Scandinavian enclaves in the Americas, Turkish areas in German towns, etc.

Adoption of plant foods and methods of cooking usually do not present any serious problems; and observations in America, Israel, and parts of Europe have shown that integration of food selections is almost complete by the second generation. Some hesitation to adopt certain animal foods may, however, persist if the particular type of food is forbidden in the home culture. The use of pork and beef is rejected by migrants from some cultures, and others demand that even permitted meat animals be slaughtered according to certain specified rituals (*shakhita, halal, jhatka*, etc). This assumes added emphasis as the average migrant worker earns more money[3] than in his home country and is able to purchase more food of animal origin than was the case before migration.

Although young age, a higher standard of education, and abilty to speak the language of the host country hasten change in food habits, they do not eliminate all difficulties, especially those stemming from religious convictions and other deep-rooted cultural influences. This has been clearly demonstrated in studies of food habits of Asian students in the United States (*17*).[4]

Various published inquiries on the food habits of migrant workers describe the methodologies used; recently, Dr Sabine Bolstorff-Bühler[5] studied the food habits of Turkish families in Berlin and developed a simple approach using in combination a questionnaire, a checklist, and interviews to gather the required information; her paper also includes an extensive bibliography.

Emigrant workers returning to their home countries take back not only hard currency and much-admired consumer goods but also newly acquired behaviour patterns, particularly food habits. The latter have not been well documented; but it is known, for example, that tea-drinking (English style, with milk and sugar) spread far and wide in rural areas of Indo-Pakistan as a result of soldiers' coming home with this habit from the two world wars. An old study of emigrants returning to southern China (Kwangtung and South Fukien) indicated that they induced an increase in the consumption of fresh fruit, which was formerly eaten only rarely, generally on festive occasions; and cold drinks (iced coffee, orange squash, etc.) became popular in a community that had traditionally consumed hot beverages (*18*).

Tourists and other transient visitors

During recent decades, the number of people who leave their homes and live elsewhere, temporarily, for reasons other than remunerative activity has increased tremendously. In 1987 their number was estimated, by the World Tourism Organization (Madrid), to be 355 million. Most of the tourists who cross international boundaries come from the industrialized countries of Europe and North America, or from Japan.

Tourists live for varying periods in hotels, boarding houses, holiday and car camps, aboard cruising ships, or other temporary habitations. Most of them are relatively affluent and in a position to demand food of their choice in the places they visit. Their choice shows two distinct trends: first, they prefer foods with which they are familiar at home, and, second, they like to try exotic and new foods, especially if presented in a form familiar to them. It has also been observed that some of the restrictions they observe at home (e.g. reduced intake of fats, carboyhydrates, and salt) tend to be disregarded during the trip, and some people consume larger quantities of food than usual – particularly in group tourism. Insufficient hygiene in some areas plus changes in patterns of food consumption increase the travellers' risk of falling ill with food-related diseases.

Pilgrims to holy places and shrines resemble tourists in several respects; but many of them differ in that they are poor, and may be subjected to overcrowded, unsanitary conditions. The incidence of gastrointestinal infections (including cholera) among them is well known. Both pilgrims and returning tourists sometimes bring back contaminants, either in their own bodies as infections or in foods intended as gifts. These have included such serious diseases as cholera, typhoid, and trichinellosis.

A taste for exotic dishes may also be brought back and passed on to family and friends, especially if these foods are marketed in the home country. By and large, however, food habits acquired during short, temporary stays abroad disappear after return to the home surroundings.

Refugees

Mass migrations of people because of war, political upheavals, and other man-made disasters have been a constant feature of human history. In recent times, millions of people have had to leave their homes, mainly in Africa and Asia, and to live in camps or other temporary colonies in neighbouring countries, which lack the necessary resources to house and feed them adequately. In spite of multinational and other help from abroad, the unfortunate refugees have to endure many kinds of deprivation.

With the exception of a few fortunate and talented people who may find jobs, most refugees have to depend on charitable common kitchens or distribution of rations. Both sources are usually deficient and result in malnutrition, especially in children. Added to the stress of misery, an uncertain future, and, sometimes, infection, the malnutrition may have serious consequences.

Rapid socioeconomic changes

An example of rapid socioeconomic change of a negative nature is the plight of refugees, mentioned above; others will be discussed under 'natural disasters'.

Positive changes, in which incomes go up and more money is available for buying food, can be illustrated by the economic developments in the Gulf countries during the last decade or so. With the increase in oil prices, economic activities and development projects suddenly increased in the 1970s, and the buying capacity of a large section of the population showed a sudden rise. As a result, importation of food of all sorts increased dramatically, the small local production achieved under difficult ecological conditions (aridity, etc.) decreased further, and imports accounted for over 95% of total consumption in some countries. The consumption of meat, eggs, poultry, fruits, dairy products, sweets, and semiprepared foods increased considerably, and that of locally caught fish and fresh desert plants decreased. The variety and choice of different types of food increased tremendously.

With the influx of a large number of foreign workers, who came mostly without their families, small restaurants and common kitchens became popular. Of course, the more affluent members of the population began to use the expensive restaurants serving international delicacies, which became prestige foods for the rest of the people.

More recently, efforts have been undertaken to increase local food production by improving agriculture through use of desalinated sea water, but this will have to be heavily subsidized in order to compete with imported foods.

Imports of large quantities of food have also created socioeconomic problems, such as the dumping of products of inferior quality or the use of ingredients that are culturally unacceptable. For example, the vast majority of people in the Gulf countries avoid blood and pork, including pork fat. Blood plasma, pork fat, or pork meat may be so intimately mixed in some foods (e.g. biscuits, pastry, sausages, etc) that it would be difficult to detect them by ordinary inspection or even by laboratory methods. The importer has to depend on the declaration of the exporter, who may or may not be strictly ethical.

Technological changes

Changes in the technology of gathering, producing, distributing, and processing food have been an important part of human development throughout the ages. They result not only from economic and cultural factors (*vide supra*) but also from acculturation and scientific advances.

The spread of food plants and animals from one part of the world to another as part of cultural exchange is well known. Even staple foods such as rice, sweet potatoes, cassava, potatoes, and maize were adopted by many societies in this way in the pre- and post-Columbian era (through the development of navigation). In recent decades improved methods of preservation and rapid means of transport have made possible the distribution of all types of food over long distances. In the richer countries one can buy foods, including fresh fruits and vegetables, from distant parts of the globe throughout the year. Preserved foods of various kinds, produced within the country or imported, are similarly available, and often are cheaper than the fresh products. The variety of prepared and semiprepared foods of local and foreign origin has increased dramatically. According to Matyas (19), the consumer in the United States now has a choice of 8000 to 12 000 food items, whereas there were only 100 or fewer items at the turn of the century.

Trends toward increasing use of convenience foods and newer methods of cooking and processing are discernible in developing countries, especially in the prosperous urban areas. The main benefit of technical advances in developing countries, however, has been the increased production of staples through the so-called green revolution. In Asia, many of the traditionally deficit countries have become self-sufficient in food. In Africa, unfortunately, these agricultural advances have not yet been fully exploited, and famines are still endemic.

Advances in food technology have also made it possible to prepare and process various kinds of food on a mass scale and to distribute them over large areas from a single plant. Similarly, methods of mass catering (20) have been developed for serving meals to large numbers of people in factories, institutions, on board ships and airplanes, etc. These developments have made home preparation of meals easier and left more time to the housewife for cultural or professional activities (21). Mass preparation of food may, however, be dangerous if the food is mishandled or the equipment is faulty or inadequately maintained.

With improvement of agriculture, the closed and non-marketing economy of rural areas changes; and farmers are able to purchase manufactured food commodities such as oils, refined sugar, and spices from outside. This change is occurring in several developing countries where rural populations, as a rule, previously consumed only locally produced food.

Apart from technological advances based on scientific progress, there is a great deal of pseudo-scientific knowledge and irrational belief that affects food behaviour. Some of this false knowledge is spread by the industry, e.g. by the manufacturers of breast-milk substitutes, 'health' foods, and alcoholic beverages. Other beliefs are spread by unscrupulous 'nutritional therapists' or 'naturists', and also by 'old wives' and similar 'wise' members of the society. Illustrations of these beliefs are the presumed invigorating effects of raw meat, milk, or fish, or the exaggerated claims made concerning the healthful properties of herbal teas or of salads made from certain wild plants. Several examples of nutrition quackery have been discussed in a monograph by the Swedish Nutrition Foundation (22).

Uncontrolled use of certain artificial fertilizers and of pesticides, anabolic and antimicrobial substances, and other agricultural chemicals that may be harmful to human health and the human environment are causing strong public reactions, especially in the industrialized countries. Some people tend to avoid foods in whose production these chemicals have been used and to demand so-called 'bio-foods'.

Other causes of changes in food behaviour

The emergency situations created by natural disasters affect the nutritional status of the population involved in a dramatic manner. Some disasters, such as severe earthquakes, volcanic eruptions, or tidal waves or floods, may cause loss of life, injuries, and tremendous loss of property, including food and means of food production. The affected population may be large, and survivors may be in a state of misery and dejection.

In other emergencies, food supplies may be primarily affected, as in seasonal or long-term drought, devastation by locusts, other forms of crop failure, or decimating animal diseases.

In disasters in which there is widespread destruction of habitations and other property, survivors are generally assembled in camps and served prepared meals from a central kitchen, at least until arrangements for alternative housing can be made. This introduces a serious food-safety problem since in this situation mass catering often has to be undertaken by people who do not know how to do it. Food contamination and microbial proliferation leading to outbreaks of food-borne diarrhoea may be the sad consequence.

Unless the afflicted country has an efficient disaster-preparedness system (which is rarely the case, even in affluent countries), there is always a delay in organizing the feeding of large numbers of people. Providing cooked meals is expensive; and even if only 'survival food' is served, this can represent a tremendous strain on the country's resources. Moreover, people quickly become bored with such meals, which generally lack variety and taste. Philanthropic organizations in industrialized countries often provide supplementary foods for disaster relief. These usually consist of powdered milk or canned foods. Frequently, these foods are unfamiliar to the affected people, who may not readily accept them. Rehabilitation may take a long time, and the survival rations may cause malnutrition, which appears first in children and other vulnerable groups, which then require supplementary feeding, sometimes of a therapeutic nature.

In parts of Africa and Asia where seasonal drought or mild, prolonged aridity is regularly experienced, people adapt to the use of wild plants and animals as a means of surviving the periods of food shortage (23). In some communities the plant foods may be supplemented by reptile and rodent meat or termites and other insects. When developing countries suffer destruction of crops by locusts, there may be a lapse of weeks or months before outside assistance arrives. People have been known to survive by feeding on wild plants (24) and on the locusts themselves, which are gathered, dried, ground, and consumed in various forms. Freedman[6] has listed food plants eaten during famine and other shortages of food in various parts of the world.

Persistent crop failures and absence of rain over long periods may cause extensive areas to become famine stricken. The situation may be complicated by the fact that the population is scattered over a large area, and may be nomadic. In such cases dry food or other rations must be distributed at designated points – water holes, former villages, etc. But even in these difficult situations, people tend to hesitate to consume unfamiliar foods. It is therefore best to obtain relief supplies within the same country or from neighbouring areas if at all possible.

Apart from emergency situations and the other factors discussed above, there are further local and personal sources of change in food behaviour. These include climatic or seasonal changes, physiological influences (e.g. puberty, pregnancy, lactation, aging), and individual factors such as a change in occupation, retirement, a high level of stress (e.g. because of the loss of a loved one), and emotional states such as grief, joy, and anger.

Interventions

Although the nutritional characteristics of human food do not change, the methods of producing, processing, and combining foods and their cultural significance change constantly under the influence of factors such as those previously discussed. Food habits are both changeable and conservative, as they are based on deeply rooted cultural traditions. The problem of a deliberate and essential quick change in food habits is very complex. What is involved in such interventions was described in some detail in 1943 by Mead (25); and in 1958, Hamburger (26) dealt with the psychological aspects. These discussions are still valid.

It is usually necessary to try to change food habits that are nutritionally deleterious and lead to malnutrition or to the transmission of agents of disease (micro-organisms, toxins, toxic chemicals, etc). The objective of the proposed change should be clearly defined. But, before deciding on an appropriate intervention and the strategies to be used, it is necessary to obtain full information about the practices to be changed – not only their health implications but also their sociocultural bases, including traditions and beliefs and economic and environmental factors.

Sometimes, current and favourite food items have to be replaced by others that are more easily obtainable (e.g. in time of war) or are nutritionally and economically advantageous. Only those habits that are significant for these or other desirable objectives should be selected for change; and care must be taken not to try to replace practices that are beneficial to, or protective of, health (e.g. thorough cooking of food and boiling of milk in warm climates) with more 'modern' technology that may require items not readily available (e.g., means of cold or hot storage, potable water, hygienic containers, etc), for economic or other reasons (27).

The Joint FAO/WHO Expert Committee on Food Safety (28) has suggested two basic criteria for intervention strategies in this area: (1) perception of the advantage of change by the community, and (2) acceptability of both the economic and the social costs. It is unrealistic to expect that an explanation of nutritional advantages alone will be perceived as such by a community. The cultural system and various beliefs about the food, or foods, concerned have to be kept in mind; and the advantage of the proposed changes should be explained to the people in terms they can understand and appreciate.

In suggesting alternatives to existing practices, one must carefully consider, in advance, the costs involved and the means of attaining the desired change. If either of these is beyond the reach of the community, cheaper and more easily available substitutes should be sought.[7] If the change involves evident economic advantages, it will, obviously, be more readily accepted.

Several cultural considerations must be borne in mind when the proposed change involves acceptance of new food items:

1. Every culture has a categorization of proper, less proper, and forbidden foods, and the people translate this into habits that become associated with taste and emotions. Total prohibition may result from religious beliefs, which should not be regarded as 'superstitions' by the health worker.

2. Unfamiliarity is one of the most frequent causes of rejection of 'new' foods. Insects, dog meat, and reptiles are rejected by many cultures, but are quite acceptable in others. Eggs, fish, and shellfish are similarly treated differently in different societies. If the aversion is not due to a religious or other strong prohibition, the unfamiliar food may become acceptable if offered in a form that resembles a familiar item.

3. Sometimes there is a physiological basis for rejection of a food. For example, an aversion to milk has been explained by a hereditary absence of lactase in the gut in certain people, and it would be futile to try to promote consumption of milk among such people.

4. The prestige value of food has a very strong influence on its acceptance or rejection. This factor should be carefully weighed and used where possible.

5. Other local conditions may determine the acceptability of certain foods. In the early days of food aid, the wheat imported into Indo-Pakistan did not have sufficient gluten to give the binding capacity to the dough that was necessary for making locally popular bread (*chapati*) and thus was not fully usable. Similarly, imported breeds of chickens were bigger than the small local breeds, but their meat was considered less tasty than the meat of the latter.

It should be borne in mind that food behaviour cannot be changed overnight, especially in peasant and tribal societies. One has to be patient and persistent. Furthermore, the road to success lies in augmenting and supplementing an existing cultural pattern, not in trying to replace it (29). It should also be realized that a change in food habits may solve only some nutrition and safety problems; others may have to be solved by approaches aimed at correcting errors and deficiencies in the food system.

Sometimes the manufacturers of food products or other commercial concerns try to induce people, through the mass media and other means, to buy and consume what they have to offer. Food-control authorities should monitor such activities carefully to ensure that they do not go against the general interests and health of the community.

Needed: a research methodology

Both for study of spontaneous changes in food habits and to evaluate the results of interventions, it is necessary to employ a systematic and uniform methodology. Studies conducted during World War 2 in some countries used methods that may still be useful in planning future investigations (see Mead & Guthe (30)). Certainly, an approach that takes cultural differences into account is essential in attempting change through health education. Wilson (31) and Fitzgerald (32), among others, have described some relevant methods that emphasize such factors.

Mead (33), in 1964, presented an outline code for describing dietary patterns that could serve as a basis for further discussion of this subject and for developing guidelines for study and comparison of food habits. She pointed out a need that still persists more than 20 years later: 'Until we construct a formal code for the recording and description of a dietary pattern, the science of food habits will remain essentially what it is today – a fragmented set of associations casually related to the relevant disciplines.'

Notes

1. I. de Garine, Food and nutrition in urban areas. Unpublished report prepared for WHO meeting on Health Consequences of Urbanization, 1970 (WHO/Recs/BHS 706). Geneva, World Health Organization.
2. This tendency is particularly strong in migrant workers in industrialized countries, who buy more expensive 'home' foods from speciality shops that have sprung up in various countries.
3. This is not always the case. Some migrant workers live in misery, especially in large towns of developing countries, and have a marginal existence.
4. H. N. Cluff, Cross cultural food problems of Iranian college students. PhD dissertation, Columbia University, New York, NY, 1963.
5. S. Bolstorff-Bühler, Verzehrsgewohnheiten   Türkischer Mitbürger in Berlin (West). Dissertation No. 142, Technische Universität, Berlin (West), 1983.
6. R. L. Freedman, Famine foods: Little known food plant resources. Unpublished manuscript, Berkeley, CA, 1972.
7. The historical anecdote of the Queen's suggesting that hungry people who cannot get bread should eat cake is liable to be repeated by agents of change of food habits.

References

1. Jelliffe, D. B., & Bennett, F. J. Cultural problems in technical assistance. *Children*, **9** (5), 171–77 (1962).
2. Kelly, I. *La antropología, la cultural y la salud pública.* Lima, Peru, Ministerio de Salud Pública y Asistencia Social, 1960.
3. Jelliffe, D. B. Social culture and nutrition. *Pediatrics*, **20** (1), 128–38.

4. Dubos, R. *Mirage of health: Utopias, progress, and biological change*. New York, Harper & Row, 1959.

5. Jelliffe, D. B., et al. The children of Hadza hunters. *Journal of Pediatrics*, **60**, 907–913 (1962).

6. Sharman, A. Nutrition and social planning. *Journal of Development Studies*, **6**, 77–91 (1970).

7. Hasan, K. A. The Hindu dietary practices and culinary rituals in a North Indian village. *Ethnomedizin*, **1**, 43–70 (1971).

8. Hendrickse, R. G. Some observations on the social background to malnutrition in tropical Africa. *African Affairs*, **65**, 341–49 (1966).

9. Cussler, M., & de Give, M. L. *'Twixt the cup and the lip: Psychological and sociocultural factors affecting food habits*. Washington, DC, Consortium Press, 1970.

10. Austin, J. E. *Confronting urban malnutrition*. Baltimore and London. Johns Hopkins University Press (for the World Bank), 1980. Pp. 3–43.

11. Velimirovič, B. Die Epidemiologie der groszstädtischen Umwelt. *Mitteilungen der Österreichischen Sanitätsverwaltung*, **76** (7–8), 2–16 (1975).

12. Thimmayama, B. V. S., Satyanarayana, K., Rao, P. K., & Swaminathan, M. C. The effect of socio-economic differences on the dietary intake of urban populations in Hyderabad. *Indian Journal of Nutrition and Dietetics*, **10**, 8–13 (1973).

13. Jelliffe, D. B., & Bennett, F. J. Different problems in different parts of the world. *Acta Paediatrica*, Suppl. 151, pp. 13–18 (1963).

14. Richards, A. I. *Land, labour and diet in northern Rhodesia. An economic study of the Bemba tribe*. London, Oxford University Press, 1951.

15. Wilson, C. S. Food taboos of childbirth: The Malay example. *Ecology of Food and Nutrition*, **2**, 267–74 (1973).

16. Foster, G. M. How to stay well in Tzintzuntzan. *Social Science and Medicine*, **19**, 523–33 (1984).

17. Ho, G. P. Factors affecting adaptation to American dietary patterns by students from the oriental countries. *Journal of Home Economics*, **58**, 277–80 (1961).

18. Chen, Ta. *Emigrant communities in South China*. New York, Institute of Pacific Relations, 1940.

19. Matyas, Z. Role of veterinarians in modern food hygiene. *Bulletin of the World Health Organization*, **56**, 699–711 (1978).

20. Charles, R. H. G. *Mass catering* (Euro Series No. 15). Copenhagen, WHO Regional Office for Europe, 1983.

21. Borgstrom, G. *Principles of food sciences*. New York, Macmillan (1968), Vol. 2, chap. 12.

22. Blix, G. (Ed.) *Food cultism and nutritional quackery* (Symposium VIII). Stockholm, Swedish Nutrition Foundation, 1970.

23. Seasonal hunger in underdeveloped countries. *Nutrition Review*, **26**, 142–45 (1968).

24. Corkhill, N. L. Dietary change in a Sudan village following locust visitation. *Africa (London)*, **19**, 1–12 (1949).

25. Mead, M. *The problem of changing food habits. Report of the Committee on Food Habits (1941–43).* Washington, DC, National Academy of Sciences, 1943.

26. Hamburger, W. W. The psychology of dietary change. *American Journal of Public Health*, **43**, 1342–48 (1958).

27. Abdussalam, M. Protective food habits. In *Proceedings of the 8th Symposium of the W.A.V.F.H., Dublin.* Dublin, World Association of Veterinary Food Hygienists, 1981. Pp. 223–30.

28. WHO Technical Report Series, No. 705, 1984 (*Food safety in health and development*: Report of the Joint FAO/WHO Expert Committee on Food Safety). Geneva, World Health Organization.

29. Niehoff, A. Changing food habits. *Journal of Nutrition Education*, Summer, pp. 10–11 (1969).

30. Mead, M., & Guthe, K. E. *Manual for the study of food habits. Report of the Committee on Food Habits.* Washington, DC, National Academy of Sciences, 1945.

31. Wilson, Ch. S. Recent methods in nutritional anthropology: Approaches and techniques. In T. K. Fitzgerald (Ed.), *Nutrition and anthropology in action.* Amsterdam, van Gorcum, 1977.

32. Fitzgerald, T. K. Anthropological approaches to the study of food habits: Some methodological issues. In T. K. Fitzgerald (Ed.), *Nutrition and anthropology in action.* Amsterdam, van Gorcum, 1977.

33. Mead, M. *Food habits research: Problems of the 1960's* (Publication No. 1225). Washington, DC, National Academy of Sciences, 1964.

3

The psychosocial environment and the development of competence in children

Theodore D. Wachs

Though poverty, malnutrition, and disease are responsible for developmental deficiences in many of the world's children, the psychological environment also plays an important role, and is often more manageable than the major physical problems. There is reason to believe that there is at least a moderate degree of continuity between the nature of a person's childhood environment and his or her behaviour as an adult. This continuity encompasses psychopathology (1–3), adjustment patterns (4), adequacy of interpersonal relationships, parenting ability (5), and general level of social functioning (6). Preventing problems in adulthood must therefore begin with helping children to cope successfully with their psychosocial environment. My focus is on that environment, on how it affects the development of *competence* in children and what we can do, preventively and therapeutically, to counter its ill effects and maximize those that are beneficial.

Why stress *competence* rather than mental health? Partly because a growing body of evidence indicates that failure to develop competence may predispose to psychopathology, rather than psychopathology lead to incompetence. Particularly relevant are studies showing a relationship between early problems in cognitive competence and later antisocial, delinquent behaviour (7–11). Another consideration is the possibility that tolerance of individual deviation stemming from mental disorder may be greater if the 'deviant' has specific skills (competences) that are valued by society (12). It has been found, for example, that training problem children in specific social skills has resulted in their being better accepted by their peers and teachers – even though the children's problem behaviours may not have changed (13). A further rationale for concentrating on the development of skills, or competences, is that this approach may make interventions more acceptable to parents who might otherwise be reluctant to seek proper treatment for their children because of the stigma associated with mental illness (14, 15).

The author is a member of the Department of Psychological Sciences, Purdue University, West Lafayette, Indiana 47907, USA.

Competence can have many meanings; it varies according to age, sex, situation, culture, and other factors (*16, 17*). Here it will refer not to *social* competence, which is culture bound, but to more general skills (*18–20*) – no value judgment being made concerning which skills may be more or less important within a particular society.

My approach, like that of Waters & Sroufe (*21*), will be developmental, focusing on skills that are most likely to help the child meet challenges from birth to adolescence. *Cognitive and interpersonal competences involve skills upon which a child can build future success; motivational competences serve to organize and promote use of appropriate skills.* The following list, derived from a much lengthier one drawn up by Anderson & Messick (*16*), presents the skills I consider particularly relevant; I have excluded categories that seemed to me to be culturally loaded.[1]

I. Cognitive competence
   1. Age-appropriate motor and perceptual skills
   2. Age-appropriate cognitive skills (i.e. language, categorization, memory, problem-solving)
   3. Flexibility in information processing and problem-solving
   4. Control of attention
   5. Appropriate curiosity and exploratory behaviour

II. Interpersonal competence
   1. Sensitivity and understanding in social and personal relationships
   2. Understanding of appropriate behaviour in different contexts
   3. Self-regulation of antisocial behaviour

III. Motivational aspects of competence
   1. Differential self-concept and realistic appraisal of self (personal worth)
   2. Understanding of self as an initiating agent in interaction with the environment
   3. Development of motivation to acquire competence (i.e. motivation to interact with and influence the environment).

The nature of environmental influences
Environment and experience
Traditional definitions of the environment refer to 'conditions, forces and external stimuli which impinge on the individual ... a network of forces which surround, engulf and play on the individual' (*23*. P. 187). Here *environment* will refer to the *objective situation*, the stimuli or response opportunities a person encounters; the aspects of the environment that actually influence the development of the child will be termed *experience*. The necessity for this distinction arises from evidence indicating that the same environment need not have the same influence on all individuals. Variations in children's reactions to the environment appear to be

mediated by specific individual characteristics of the organism. This phenomenon has been termed *organismic specificity* (24).

The impact of the environment on the child's development can be mediated by many factors. Among them is sex, and a number of studies have detailed its effects, particularly in the early years (24). Studies have revealed differences, for example, in the reactivity of males and females to parental agreement on rearing practices (25), quality of day care (26), school environments (27, 28), stress (5, 29, 30), and spacing of sibs (31).

Another organismic factor that predisposes to differences in reactivity is *biological vulnerability*. There is evidence suggesting greater sensitivity to stress in children who are especially vulnerable because of parental psychopathology (32–34) or antisocial behaviour (35). Studies (36, 38), primarily of infants, have also suggested that a child's *temperament* and activity level (39–40) may mediate his reaction to his environment: common to both these areas is evidence indicating that infants having either biomedical vulnerability or a difficult temperament seem to have a narrower range of response to the environment than do those with an easy temperament (41, 42). Other organismic characteristics that appear to mediate relationships between environment and development include *intelligence* (27, 37, 43–45), *race* (46, 47), and qualities such as *self-regulation, energy level*, and *stimulus-control capacities* (37).

The transitional nature of environmental influences

The long-held view that early experiences have a virtually unchangeable impact on later development has been challenged by the Clarkes and co-workers (48, 49), who maintain that although early experience is relevant for development, its importance is primarily a function of being part of a developmental process. The available evidence does suggest, however, that some long-term effects of early experiences are independent of intervening environments (47, 50–52); there also appears to be some agreement that experiences occurring earlier in life may have a greater impact than those in later life (5, 24, 53).

It is also agreed, however, that, rather than thinking in terms of critical periods in development, it is better to conceive of the relationship of environment to development as a *process* involving both early and later experiences. For example, it has been found that the impact of early institutionalization on development can be mediated by the quality of the environment the child encounters after release from the institution (51, 52, 54). Studies of family environments (55–57) and of interventions attempted after infancy (53, 58) also support the concept of environment as process.

The transactional nature of the environment

The environment–development influence has been shown to be bidirectional (59, 60): in a multistage temporal process, the environment may initially influence the child, but the child will in turn influence the resulting environment, which in turn will subsequently influence the child. Empirical research has suggested a number of possible characteristics of the child that may be particularly influential in altering the environment, including intelligence (61, 62), prematurity (42), malnutrition (63–65), and temperament (66). It has also been hypothesized that the critical factor in a child's influence on his environment may be not the child's characteristics *per se* as much as the match between those characteristics and caregiver behaviours, perceptions, and values (38).

The structure of the environment

Bronfenbrenner (67) has distinguished four levels of the environment, each lower level being nested within a higher level, like a set of Russian dolls. The highest level is the *macrosystem*, which involves cultural patterns and ecology. Nested within the macrosystem is the *exosystem*, which refers to both formal (e.g. government institutions) and informal (e.g. social support networks) social structures. Nested within the exosystem is the *mesosystem*, which refers to interactions among institutions, individuals, and settings. Nested under the mesosystem is the *microsystem*, which refers to the family, or to children's interactions with their parents. Differences have been distinguished within each of these levels as well. For example, in the microsystem, distinctions have been made between stimuli and responses (68), *within* versus *between* family environments (69), and physical and social environments (24, 70).

A number of investigators (67, 71–78) have pointed out that parental influences at the microsystem level may be shaped or reinforced, at least to some extent, by ecological or cultural pressures emanating from higher levels of the system. For example, in situations in which there is a clash between religious and political cultures (79), there may be active resistance at the microsystem level to influences from higher levels in the system.

Other studies indicate that ecological, social, and cultural factors from higher levels of the system appear to *mediate* the relationship of environment to aggressive behaviour (80, 81), the process of socialization (82), the development of internal controls (83) the development of child psychopathology (84, 85), children's academic achievement and attitudes toward school (44, 86), the development of imaginative play in children (87), and the impact of crowding (88, 89).

Thus, though variations in behaviour due to the environment may be primarily a function of the microsystem, the influences of that system are themselves shaped by higher-level factors within the system. The data therefore suggest that environment–development relationships at the microsystem level may be of *limited generalizability,* because of influences from other levels of the environment. At the very least, this means that great care must be taken in trying to transfer intervention programmes developed in one culture to other cultures.

Specificity of environmental action

As both Hunt (*90, 91*) and Wachs (*92, 93*) have noted, environment–development relationships have generally been treated in a global fashion – that is, it has been assumed that an environment could be characterized as either good or bad, and that good environments facilitated, and bad environments impeded, all aspects of development. The available evidence (*24, 93*) suggests, however, that specific aspects of development will be influenced *only* by specific aspects of the environment. This phenomenon is called *environmental specificity.* Environmental specificity means that, from a practical standpoint, no environment may be totally good or totally bad. A specific set of environmental qualities may facilitate the development of a certain set of skills, be irrelevant in the development of another, and hinder the development of a third set of skills.

At the level of the macrosystem, for example, Elder (*43*) found that growing up during a depression lowered children's self-esteem, but increased their sense of responsibility and their industriousness. Several studies (*94, 95*) have shown that being reared in isolated settings has a detrimental impact on the development of competence in interpersonal relationships, but has little effect on the development of cognitive skills.

At the exosystem level, the available data include that schooling does not result in a uniform increase in all cognitive skills, but in only those involving abstract or hypothetical thinking or mental manipulation (*96*). Moreover, different patterns of teacher behaviour within schools appear to be associated with differences in the cognitive development of their pupils (*97*).

The specificity of microsystem environmental influences had been repeatedly demonstrated in relation to the development of cognitive (*98–102*) and language (*103*) skills and other areas of functioning. Recent studies indicate that parent–child separation caused by divorce tends to be correlated with acting-out behaviours in children, whereas separation caused by death of a parent tends to give rise to anxious, withdrawn behaviour (*29, 104, 105*). The effects also vary according to whether the loss is of the mother or the father (*106*). Differences in the impact of environmental influences on child personality (*107*), psychopathology (*108*), antisocial behaviour (*2*), and adolescent drug use (*109*) have also been reported.

Environment as covariate

The environment does not act in isolation, but rather covaries with a variety of other influences that can also affect development. Empirically, one of the most consistent findings in the literature involves the covariance of an adverse psychosocial environment with malnutrition (110–115). For example, Craviotto & Delicardie (116) found that the homes of malnourished children offered significantly less environmental stimulation before and after the malnutrition episode than did the homes of adequately nourished children. A similar covariance pattern is observed in the relation between the quality of the child's psychosocial environment and the likelihood of his suffering disease or biological insult (50, 60, 117–119), or between genetic and environmental factors in the etiology of mild mental retardation (120) and behavioural competence (121).

One implication of such findings is that the greater the degree of covariance, the greater the psychological risk to the child. For instance, Sameroff & McDonough (122), using an additive risk score, reported a significant linear relationship between the number of biosocial risks a child encountered and measures of either cognitive or interpersonal competence: as the number of biosocial risks impinging on the child increased, the child's scores on cognitive or interpersonal competence measures decreased. In contrast, the impact of a single biological or social risk factor appeared to be fairly limited. Similar findings have been reported by Rutter (5, 105) and by Werner & Smith (30).

What this means in practice is that when a child is at psychosocial risk because of economic disadvantage, one must be extremely cautious in attributing behavioural deficits *primarily* to environmental factors: the deficits could also be due to biomedical factors that covary with an inadequate environment. The converse also holds true, however: in situations in which children are at biomedical risk, great care must be exercised in attributing behavioural deficits *primarily* to biomedical factors, since those deficits could just as easily be associated with covarying environmental factors (123).

The obvious implication is that, in working with child populations at risk, both biomedical and environmental factors must be considered in planning interventions (124). To the extent that the environment covaries with biomedical problems and *is relevant to the behaviour under study*, the impact of intervention will be magnified if both biomedical and environmental components are included in the intervention process.

Specific environmental factors at different levels and the development of competence

The macrosystem level

Cognitive competence

Except for a study suggesting that isolation from the mainstream of a culture, as evidenced by the use of a dialect at home, may be related to poor cognitive outcomes (125), little recent data are available on the relationship of macro-environmental factors to the development of cognitive competence in children since a review by Graham in 1977 (126). However, there has been an increasing interest in what may be called the development of *cognitive style parameters*, such as *field independence* versus *field dependence* (whether the person uses an internal or an external frame of reference in dealing with the environment), and *psychological differentiation* (the complexity and integration of behaviour patterns a person displays).

Witkin & Berry (78) have presented a compelling body of evidence suggesting that the development of cognitive styles is a function of both the natural ecology and the social structure associated with that ecology. Specifically, ecologies that lead to hunter–gatherer life-styles, requiring independence and self-reliance, are found to be associated with the development of field independence and high differentiation. Ecological settings that predispose to agricultural life-styles, requiring cooperation, social sensitivity, and the development of social controls, are found to be associated with field dependence and lower levels of differentiation. On the basis of a survey of 17 cultures, Berry (71) reports that knowledge of culture and ecology alone enables one to predict about 50% of the variability in cognitive styles. A lower, though still significant, prediction rate is found *within cultures*. Berry notes that this relationship holds primarily for subsistence societies; as acculturation increases, the relevance of ecological factors for cognitive style seems to decrease.

Interpersonal and motivational competence

In his 1977 review (126), Graham related a number of cultural factors to interpersonal and motivational development, including patterns of aggression within cultures and degree of urbanization.

Across a variety of cultures, urbanization and industrialization have been implicated as causing a reduction in family interactions, increased intergenerational conflict, and inadequate socialization of children (127–129). The consequent effects on children (according to clinical observations) for the most part include increased drug abuse (130, 131), increased vulnerability to behavioural problems (127), loss of a sense of personal control, a decrease in delay of gratification (132), and an increase in adolescent identity confusion (131, 133). There is, however, some evidence that the impact of urbanization may be mediated by the child's perception of the urban environment (134) and by previous cultural patterns, such as the degree of contact of the father with his children in a traditional society (135).

Recent data on the influence of cultural factors on children's adjustment deal particularly with the impact of violent cultures, as characterized by the frequency of wars, revolutions, or terrorist activities. Although children seem to be affected primarily during acute phases of fighting (136), by-products of cultural violence, such as forced migration, do appear to be associated with an increased sense of learned helplessness in children (115). What is most notable, however, is the tremendous resilience displayed by children in the face of major cultural disruptions, such as war (137).

A number of factors may mediate the child's reaction to cultural violence. Environmental buffering factors included level of social support (*138*) and the quality of parental reactions (*137*). Individual (organismic) characteristics may also be important. For example, data from Israel (*139*) indicate that the impact of paternal death in battle seems especially salient for male children, who are characterized as having lower levels of social adjustment, striving for achievement and independence, higher levels of aggression, and more peer problems. In contrast, the impact on girls seems more positive in terms of higher levels of independence and social assertiveness. These data are particularly critical in that the findings do not appear to be confounded by either economic stress or differential maternal treatment.

The direct impact of cultural violence on children's own aggressive behaviour is not yet clear. Studies of children living in Northern Ireland report contradictory results: McWhirter & Trew (*140*) found surprisingly little impact on children growing up in the midst of violence, whereas Fields (*141*) concluded that children who were victims of violence grew up to be violent adults.

More work in this area is needed. Two approaches might be useful in future research:

1. The adaptive-cost model (*88, 142*) postulates that there is a cost associated with people's adaptation to difficult situations such as cultural violence. This model suggests the need for long-term follow-up of children who have been exposed to violence to determine the cost of their adaptation.
2. Determination of the factors that discriminate between children who transcend the impact of cultural violence and those who are adversely affected by it might distinguish more precisely which factors might serve as buffers (*30*).

The exosystem level

Cognitive competence

In his review Graham (*126*) noted the relevance of school influences, school attendance being associated with higher levels of cognitive competence in children. Subsequent reviews and research seem, with certain reservations, to confirm that conclusion (*96, 125, 143, 144*). There is, of course, tremendous variability among schools in terms of their impact on children (*143, 145*), which raises the question of which characteristics of individual schools are most likely to promote the development of cognitive competence.

Within minimal limits, for both preschools (*146*) and primary and secondary schools (*145*), factors such as physical facilities, number of books in the library, school size, and amount of money spent per pupil do *not* appear to relate to academic achievement. What does appear to be relevant are what might be called

expectancy parameters, such as an orientation toward achievement within the school
(*145*), or student perceptions of the school as cohesive, organized, and goal
directed (*44*). Also relevant are organizational factors such as regularity in requiring
and marking homework and teacher time spent actually teaching, not maintaining
order and discipline. Good class structure and sensitivity to students, as evidenced
in feedback to students and rewards for good performance, also seem to be
important (*145*).

Another exosystem factor is the social support networks available to the
family – persons outside the immediate home who are available to help the family,
directly or indirectly (*147*). Recent data indicate a better cognitive outcome at four
years of age for biomedically at-risk infants whose mothers had social supports
available to them; this is particularly true for lower-class mothers (*148*). Earlier
research yielded conflicting evidence on whether social support resulted in better
rearing environments (*149, 150*). More recent studies have indicated that whether
social support is translated into better rearing environments depends on both
exosystem factors (mothers whose husbands' work takes them away from the home
community have fewer support networks, which in turn relates to less-adequate
rearing patterns [*72*]) and on *child characteristics* (the association between support
and sensitive parent rearing is found only for parents of irritable infants [*151*]).

Interpersonal and motivational competence

School has a socializing as well as a cognitive influence on the child (*152*). The most
rapid cultural change has been observed to occur where there are few transmitters
and many recipients (*153*), a situation that typifies the school in terms of ratio of
teachers to pupils. The available evidence suggests that socialization within the
schools occurs most rapidly under conditions of homogeneity of social setting (*77*),
central control of reinforcements, reward of compliance and non-compliance not
being rewarded, use of multiple, high-status, social models who support each other,
and a definite group status that relates to age (*152*).

It should be noted that we are assuming agreement between the school and
traditional cultural settings, such as the family, in terms of the values to be
socialized. Particularly in developing countries, a number of observers have
commented on the difficulties encountered when schools promote such values as
independence, self-reliance, and critical thinking (*115*) while the homes promote
convergent thought, dependence on the family, and cooperative behaviour. Such
conditions may lead to parent–child conflict (*129, 154*).

Moreover, although it seems clear that schools can have a facilitating impact on
certain dimensions of cognitive competence, a cautionary note has been sounded
by clinicians in developing countries: because of the tremendous competition for
a limited number of places in higher grades, school-age children in these countries
may be subjected to high levels of stress and family pressure (*155, 156*), and a
child's failure to meet family achievement demands may have a negative impact on

the child (128, 156). In such situations schooling may be a mixed blessing for some children.

School attendance has been found to be associated with a variety of other interactional and motivational competencies, depending on the nature of the school environment. It can, for instance, reduce delinquency (145), enhance self-esteem (145, 157), and increase motivation to achieve academically (145, 158). Of particular interest are studies suggesting that the development of a sense of internalized responsibility in students is associated with schools that promote students' self-direction of their learning experiences (159) and grant them both more privileges and more responsibilities (160). In contrast, schools that discourage pupil initiative and active pupil involvement in school affairs promote a feeling of learned helplessness (161). The generalizability of such data may, however, be limited by cultural factors (83).

There are few data on the influence of institutions other than the schools on the development of interpersonal and motivational competence in children. Studies of adults suggest that social support networks may serve as a buffer against stress (105, 162); and clinical data indicate that the extended family may serve the same purpose for children (128). This is still a relatively uncharted area, however.

The microsystem level
Cognitive competence

Much of the available information on the microsystem and cognitive development during the first five years of life has been reviewed by Wachs & Gruen (24), and is summarized in Table 1.

A meta-analysis of a number of major longitudinal studies (163) and other research investigations (46, 56, 164–169) have confirmed the relevance of parental involvement, variety of stimulation, responsivity of the environment, and language stimulation for both cognitive performance and later academic achievement. Other factors that have been shown to be related to various aspects of early cognitive functioning include sensitivity (164), early tactile stimulation (169), and direct skills teaching (148).

Recent data confirmed the time-limited influence of early bonding experience on subsequent cognitive development (170, 171) and have pointed out the relevance for both enhanced early cognitive development (93) and subsequent school achievement (172) of older siblings' verbal interactions with younger sibs.

Parental values and direct parental interaction have been noted to be important for the cognitive development of school-age children and adolescents (173). A review by Seginer (174) reports that 9 of 11 studies indicate a positive relationship between parental achievement values and children's actual achievement, a relationship that seems to hold across cultures. Similar results have been reported in a number of other studies (99, 175–177). Witkin (178) found that, in terms of

Table 1. *Summary of environmental factors showing consistent relationships to cognitive development over the first five years of life*

Parameters	Direction of relationship to cognitive performance	Comments
I. Physical environmental parameters		
Availability of stimulus	Positive	Primarily relevant in first nine months of life
Variety of stimulus	Positive	As child gets older, changes in available objects may be more critical than number of different objects available
Responsivity of the physical environment	Positive	
Ambient background noise	Negative	Particularly salient for males and at-risk infants
Overcrowding	Negative	
Regularity of scheduling	Positive	May be mediated by age and by ability under study
Physical restraints on exploration	Negative	
II. Social environmental parameters		
Amount of parent/child interaction	Positive	Consistent relationship does not appear until second year of life
Tactual kinesthetic stimulation	Positive	Primarily salient between birth and 6 months of age
Contingent responses to child	Positive	Specificity in salience of different types of contingencies at different ages
Sensitivity to child cues	Positive	
Verbal stimulation	Positive	Salient primarily only after 12 months of age
Parental restrictions on exploration	Negative	
Direct skill teaching by parent	Positive	
III. Interpersonal environmental parameters		
Emotional warmth	Positive	Mediated by high levels of specificity
Controlling orientation	Negative	

cognitive style, families valuing independence of action had children who tended to be field independent, whereas parents who valued conformity had children who tended to be field dependent. This, too, appears to hold within and across cultures.

Active parental involvement or guidance facilitates older children's cognitive development (52, 100, 175) and academic achievement (62), and has been stressed in successful intervention projects (53). Other positive influences are the variety of intellectually stimulating materials in the home (100) and direct language training of the child (175) (the latter may be generalizable only in Western cultures [62]).

Certain aspects of family structure seem also to influence cognitive development (44, 179–182), among them absence of the father, which has consistently been reported to have a negative impact (102). It is still unclear, however, whether this relationship is due to the loss of paternal involvement with the child, increased family stress associated with the father's absence (102), or the change in socioeconomic status that often follows loss of the father (183).

A final environmental factor that appears to be salient for the cognitive functioning of older children is peer-group educational aspirations. A review of the literature (184) has indicated a modest but consistent impact of peer-group aspirations, higher aspirations being associated with higher achievement. This influence appears to be particularly strong for those living in urban settings.

Interpersonal and motivational competence

The Wachs & Gruen review (24) covers microsystem influences, over the first five years of life, for the development of interpersonal and motivational competence. The findings are summarized in Table 2.

In addition to the data reported in Table 2, infant exploratory behaviour has been found to be positively related to parental attention-focusing behaviours (pointing, demonstration) (185), but negatively related to maternal prohibitions (186). Similarly, the degree of impulse control shown by toddlers has been found to be negatively related to the amount of physical punishment utilized by parents (187). Persistence in problem-solving tasks at 13 months has been reported to be positively related to six-month measures of the amount of kinesthetic and auditory stimulation, amount of adult mediation of the child's play, number of available responsive toys (188), and variety of stimulation (165). A recent study (189) notes a high degree of environmental and organismic specificity in the relationship between environment and mastery behaviour in infancy.

In the preschool period, maternal involvement has been found to facilitate the development of a sense of internalized responsibility (190, 191). Parental encouragement of the child's social maturation and parental avoidance of physical punishment have a positive relationship to the development of self-reliance. The availability of intellectually stimulating objects in the home promotes the child's showing initiative in the classroom (192).

Table 2. *Summary of microsystem parameters that relate to the development of indices of interpersonal competence over the first five years*

Parameters	Direction of relationship	Comments
Early stress (institutionalization, separation, family discord)	Negative	Primarily for very early stress
Responsive environment	Positive	
Increasing dyadic interaction between mother and child (fit between mother and infant behaviour)	Positive	Primarily after 12 months of age. This appears to be a system process in which mothers become more effective at correctly recognizing cues and responding appropriately and the child utilizes the feedback to alter his/her behaviour
Authoritative parent rearing style (controlling but warm and receptive to child's communications and problems)	Positive	May be mediated by sex of the child
Direct parental teaching of socialization skills and rationales	Positive	May be mediated by sex of child. Choice of disciplinary strategy may also be mediated by the child's characteristics and situational factors
Father's absence	Negative	Impact particularly salient during first five years of life. Impact may be buffered by the presence of alternative male models and mediated by the reasons for the father's absence

For older children, Graham (*126*) has noted the relevance of separation, family discord, quality of parental supervision, and parental disciplinary practices. Absence of the father has been shown to be related to lower levels of ego strength and self-confidence in children (*193*). However, there is no consensus among researchers concerning the relationship between separation from the father and aggressive behaviour in children or later adult criminality (*2, 194–196*). A major review of this topic (*29*) suggests a time-limited relationship between separation and behaviour problems.

In contrast, both reviews and longitudinal research studies have consistently implicated family discord as a major etiological factor in the production of antisocial behaviour, aggression, and delinquency in children (5, 7, 9, 29, 197). The impact of family discord appears particularly strong for crimes against persons (2), and this relationship seems to hold across cultures (29). Family discord has also been implicated as a cause of various non-clinical behaviour problems in children across several cultures (11, 84, 198), and to be related to maladaptive behaviour in the classroom (199, 200) and to low social status (9). On the other hand, family cohesiveness has been found to predict adolescents' task persistence and conscientiousness (201) and children's ability to cope with their environment and with internal stress (37). A growing body of evidence suggests that disturbances in family communication may relate to child psychopathology (202) (particularly in terms of a breakdown when there is a genetic risk [108, 203]) *and to peer ratings of the child in terms of interpersonal competence (204).*

Harsh parental punishment, rejection of the child, and inconsistent discipline may predispose to antisocial, aggressive, and delinquent behaviour on the part of the child (2, 7), particularly when the child is young and is not well identified with the parent (9). This relationship appears in both Western and non-Western societies (155). Given this pattern of evidence, it is perhaps not surprising that toddlers who have been abused by their parents show the same patterns of behaviour toward distressed peers that their abusing parents have displayed towards them (205). The effects of physical punishment may, however, be tempered by whether or not the child perceives the parent as caring for him or her (37). Poor supervision of the child may also have a deleterious influence (2, 7). Parental attitudes may also be a buffering factor, given evidence indicating that parental acceptance of the child may lead to lower rates of recidivism following arrest for delinquency (206).

Besides predicting interpersonal behaviour, microsystem factors have also been shown to be related to specific motivational competencies. The child's development of an internalized sense of responsibility has been found to be positively related to the mother's stressing responsibility in achievement (83), whereas maternal restrictions on child-initiated actions lead to an externalized sense of responsibility (207). This seems to confirm findings that parental encouragement of the child's independence produces greater striving for independence in the child (201). The development of achievement motivation in children has been shown to be related to the degree to which their parents use contingent rewards (reward or punishment contingent on the child's action) (73) and to the availability and warmth of the parent (208).

As for peers as an environmental influence, exposure to non-delinquent peers appears to reduce chances of recidivism in delinquent boys (206); and exposure to non-retarded peers promotes higher levels of social competence in retarded children (209).

The environment as buffer

Genetic risks

Much of the available evidence confirming the role of the environment as a buffer against genetic deficits comes from studies of infants or children with Down's syndrome. It has been found that intellectual gains or losses experienced by these children are directly related to the type of rearing environment to which they are exposed (*169, 210–212*). Moreover, early intervention programmes with infants and preschoolers with Down's syndrome have reported significant gains in cognitive functioning (*213, 214*). For example, Down's syndrome children who had been exposed to an environmental enrichment programme for the first six years of life had school-age IQ scores in the 80s and were able to read at primary-grade level (*215*).

In areas other than cognitive competence, the majority of offspring of schizophrenic parents show essentially normal development. The available data indicate that at least part of the variance associated with such children's 'invulnerability' is environmental in nature (*216–218*). For example, a relationship with either a disturbed or a non-disturbed parent that is characterized by availability and parental warmth can serve as a buffer for a child at genetic risk for schizophrenia (*208*). Similarly, the risk of criminality for children whose fathers were criminals has been found to be reduced by adoption into non-criminal families (*219*). Early intervention in the form of a nursery-school programme beginning at age three has also been shown to reduce the risk of later psychosis or antisocial behaviour (*220*). Even the self-mutilative behaviour associated with the Lesch-Nyhan syndrome has been reported to respond to a programme involving increasing adult attention to non-mutilative behaviour and concomitant decreasing attention to attempts at self-mutilation (*221*).

Biomedical risk

Evidence of the role of the environment in buffering the effects of pre- or peri-natal biomedical insults (e.g. prematurity, postmaturity, respiratory distress) is provided by studies (*60, 222, 223*) suggesting more favourable outcomes for at risk infants from 'higher social-class groups'. Research utilizing more detailed measures of home environments of biomedically at risk children also supports this conclusion (*224–227*). For example, longitudinal data indicate that pre-term infants with EEG patterns indicative of problems in central nervous system organization are at significant risk for cognitive impairment at eight years of age. However, if these at risk infants are reared in attentive, responsive, home environments, their cognitive performance is found to be above average at eight years (*228*). Environmental intervention studies with at risk populations provide further evidence of buffering effects (*229–237*).

Although most of the available evidence deals with infants, there are also data indicating gains in both cognitive (238, 239) and interpersonal (240) skills from either psychosocial interventions or appropriate home environments (241) with older moderately or severely organically retarded children.

Malnutrition, a common risk factor in many parts of the world, has been shown to respond better to nutritional treatment plus environmental intervention than to supplemental nutrition alone (115). For instance, an intervention study of foetally malnourished infants by Zeskind & Ramey (65, 242) demonstrated that the infants who received special day-care environmental intervention were indistinguishable in cognitive or interpersonal functioning from non-malnourished controls, whereas infants receiving standard medical care alone displayed deficits in cognitive and interpersonal performance through at least three years of age. The relevance of the environment as a buffer, and of the principle of environmental specificity, has been shown in studies of other malnourished populations as well (64, 112, 243–245).

As Sigman (124) has noted, one major implication of the finding that the environment can be a significant buffer against risk conditions is that maximal development is promoted when interventions for biomedically at risk children include environmental as well as medical components.

Psychosocial risk

Psychosocial risk is not well defined, but typically involves children living in home environments that foster the development of mild mental retardation – it being understood, of course, that the retardation can be due to the impact of either social or biological factors. Attempts at intervention have been shown to minimize the risk of mild retardation in this population (246–248). Moreover, there is evidence that the interventions have had a beneficial effect on the mothers in addition to the children, increasing their participation in community affairs (249), or encouraging them to resume their formal education (250).

Buffering effects have been shown to extend beyond cognitive skills. Hunt (251), studying the impact of a language stimulation programme on institutionalized infants in Iran, reported higher levels of social interaction and more positive emotional expressiveness in the infants involved in the programme. Older children at risk for behaviour disorders because of loss of a parent or family antisocial behaviour or discord have responded favourably to such environmental buffers as exposure to surrogate parents (252), extended-family influences (3), and attendance at high-quality schools (57).

Multiple risks

Data dealing directly with the question of whether the environment can play a buffering role against multiple risks are sparse, but a seminal study by Werner & Smith (30) provides an affirmative answer. Their results indicate that a complex network of factors appears to produce 'vulnerable' or 'invulnerable' children and that psychological factors are critical:

> Among key factors in the care giving environment that appear to contribute to the resiliency and stress resistance of these high risk children were: the age of the opposite sex parent (younger mothers for resilient males, older fathers for resilient females); the number of children in the family (4 or fewer); the spacing between the index child and the next sibling (more than two years); the number and type of alternative caretakers available within the household (father, grandparents, older siblings); the work load of the mother (including steady employment outside of the household); the amount of attention given to the child by the primary caretakers in infancy; the availability of a sibling as a caretaker or confidante in childhood; structure and rules in the household in adolescence; cohesiveness of the family; the presence of an informal multigenerational network of kin and friends in adolescence. (Pp. 154–55)

Congruent with the notion of the cumulative nature of environmental action, some buffering factors were found to be associated uniquely with infancy whereas others were important in childhood or adolescence. The data also suggest the possibility of organismic specificity in terms of the child's sex and temperament affecting outcome.

Interventions and their impact
In terms of intervention, discussion of projects that have been reported to be successful in Western industrialized societies will be minimal since, because of their cost and cultural factors, they are unlikely to be practical in other settings. Examples of such projects can be found elsewhere (250, 253–257).

Principles of intervention
In light of the large numbers of children who appear to need behavioural intervention (8), a number of researchers have stressed the following steps: (1) the importance of identifying children who are at high risk for specific problems and directing intervention toward those children; (2) developing specific interventions for particular goals (24, 120, 250, 258, 259). There is increasing agreement that in both early (260) and later (44) interventions it is critical to take into account the individual characteristics of the children who are to be involved. Further, it is my belief that to be maximally effective, intervention must be based on known principles of environmental action rather than on theoretical speculation about what should work. Thus, strategies employed should be based on demonstrated empirical relationships between specific competencies and specific environmental parameters as described in the previous sections.

Ramey and co-workers (250) have also stressed that focusing on just one layer of the environment is apt to produce only limited gains, and that one should intervene at points at which one can have maximal impact within the whole system. Since environmental action is best conceived of as a process, a single, time-limited intervention is less likely to produce long-term gains than a continuing series of interventions, each building upon previous gains (58, 182). Moreover, given that children are more likely to encounter multiple rather than single stresses (5, 122) and that behaviour is determined by a multitude of factors, intervention should be multidimensional, focusing simultaneously on a number of biosocial elements (167).

Intervention at the macrosystem level

It has been pointed out that, for a variety of reasons, recommendations concerning interventions often wind up being buried in files or stored in dusty warehouses rather than being implemented, by programme planners (261). Why are recommendations often not implemented? First, there is the matter of political feasibility. Planners may be more than willing to issue policy statements about the importance of intervention programmes; but unless cost-effective gains are seen as emerging from such interventions, they are not likely to be translated into social action (115). Second, the extent to which intervention programmes contradict popular folk beliefs appears to be inversely related to the likelihood of their being accepted and implemented by the target population (261). For instance, parent – child interaction patterns that are seen by parents as having functional utility are not likely to be replaced, regardless of how many detrimental consequences of those patterns outside experts may point to (76). It is only when parents see interventions as a more functional alternative to what is currently being done that they are likely to accept and participate in them.

What is common to both these factors is the necessity of convincing two distinct groups – politicians and parents – of the importance of psychosocial intervention. There is obviously no universal way to achieve this; one possibility is use of the mass media, particularly television and radio, which are becoming increasing influences even in developing countries (262). Information directed at those who make and implement policy should focus on the cost effectiveness of intervention programmes for children, in terms of both potential future productivity and national pride. Information directed at parents could include guidance on viable alternatives to traditional child-rearing practices. Examples of informational programmes that can be used in this way have been given in a paper by McCall, Gregory, & Murray (263).

Use of the mass media as an instrument of social change is an extremely complex business, but one point seems clear: programme content must be developed within the specific culture and be tied to existing realities in that culture rather than be imposed from outside (264).

Intervention at the exosystem level

At the level of the exosystem, the factor most often emphasized in recent literature is the need for social support networks. The formation of support networks has been proposed as a means of replacing the loss of the extended family or tribe in cultures undergoing rapid social change (*132, 265*). Researchers have pointed out the impossibility of training mothers to intervene effectively with their children when the mothers have to deal continually with major social or interpersonal crises; the use of support networks to buffer mothers against these crises is stressed as a necessary first step in the intervention process (*148, 266*).

Professionals may function here either in training health-care workers to identify and strengthen existing support networks for families in which there are children at risk, or in developing community-based support networks where none exist.

Adoption

One radical possibility for exosystem intervention involves the suggestion that mechanisms be set up for early adoption into high-quality environments of either unwanted children (*126*) or children living with their biological parents in environments that are detrimental to the development of competence (*267*). Obviously, it would be best if the biological parents could be worked with through community support and direct intervention to change the nature of the child's environment; but in situations in which improvement has been tried and failed, the evidence suggests that adoption into a better setting, *within the child's culture*, may be a more humane step than allowing the child to remain with its biological parents in a detrimental environment.

Some quite dramatic results have been observed in adoption studies in which children, born into backgrounds that predispose to cognitive impairment, have been adopted early in life by families that could provide more adequate environmental stimulation than the children would have normally received (*45, 268, 269*). Moreover, the impact of adoption into better home environments extends beyond just cognitive competence. Bohman & Sigvardsson (*54*) have reported significantly better behaviour among children of antisocial or alcoholic parents who were adopted into more normal home environments, noting that the quality of the environment into which the child is adopted seems critical.

Institutions and alternatives

Decrements in competence associated with institutional rearing (*209, 270, 271*) can be attributed to either stimulus deprivation, or to the fact that less-competent children are the ones who have been institutionalized. However, the evidence from attempts at environmental intervention with institutionalized infants (*6, 272–274*) and studies of older, institutionalized, retarded children (*239*) indicate either gains in cognitive functioning or arrest of the decline in functioning associated with institutional rearing. Moreover, the degree of decrement appears to be a function of the adequacy of environmental stimulation provided by the institution (*275,*

276): if the institution offers adequate stimulation, institutionalized children may show higher levels of cognitive performance than children reared by their biological parents in inadequate home environments (276).

Both the cost of institutionalization (8) and the problems associated with its psychological effects (277) have led to a search for alternatives to institutional care. But since the severity of the child's condition or family or culture pressures may make institutionalization unavoidable, attention must be paid to making institutions more stimulating and healthful.

As Mortimore (278) has pointed out, within certain minimal limits, physical aspects are much less critical than quality and number of staff. Ideally, staff should be trained in many of the environmental principles discussed here. Even a limited staff may be enabled to provide more than custodial care, if its members are permitted a measure of autonomy in child-care decisions and some flexibility in use of their time within the institution.

One alternative to institutions is what are known as 'therapeutic villages': children being placed in group homes within a normal village setting (277). The treatment gains in these settings may occur either as a direct function of specific cognitive (53) or behavioural (279) training experiences, or as a result of the children's exposure to normal children who have higher levels of social competence (209) or who can serve as non-delinquent role models (206). Often such direct training and exposure facilitate each other, as when delinquent children are trained in interpersonal skills that enable them to interact more effectively with non-delinquent children (206). This type of setting may be particularly useful for children who have been abandoned, or for those whose behaviour is so deviant that people in their home milieu have difficulty accepting and coping with them.

Another alternative to institutionalization would be the development of community centres within a child's home village. Such centres could function in a variety of ways. They could act as clearing houses for the development and dissemination of resources within the community (267). They could also be used for day-care programmes, providing early cognitive interventions that might serve as a buffer for infants who have been identified as being at risk for future mental retardation (280). Finally, for older children with antisocial or behavioural problems, centre personnel could develop appropriate behaviour-change programmes (281).

Schools

The setting with the most potential for acting as a focus for intervention, *but that is the most underused at present*, is the school (287). As has been noted earlier, schools can serve as environmental buffers for children (5). This is particularly true if the school stresses high achievement expectations, provides positive feedback to the children, allows them to assume responsibility within the school system, adequately manages discipline problems, and avoids physical punishment as a means of dealing with educational or behaviour problems (5, 267, 283).

By being sensitive to what parents in the community will accept, the school can increase the degree of parental involvement with the school, and thus help to intergrate micro- and exo-system influences in specific problem areas (44). Programmes for enhancing cognitive skills in disadvantaged school-age children are an example of this approach. In one such programme the school provided parents with both materials and information on how to work effectively with their children, and the parents pledged to stress achievement values and to reward their children's gains (284). Other programmes have involved joint parent and school efforts to change problem behaviours. Typically, the schools define what behaviours are appropriate and provide daily feedback to parents on whether their children have met behavioural expectations; on the basis of the school reports, the parents then provide appropriate rewards or punishments for the children at home (285).

The use of schools as a means of enhancing children's competence has generally involved only those old enough to attend school. However, as Zigler & Finn (267) have pointed out, there is no reason why the school cannot extend its influence downward to serve preschool-age children and even infants. In coordinated efforts with community centres, schools could act both as diagnostic centres, identifying young children at risk for cognitive impairment, and as resources centres for parents concerned about their children's development. Involving the school directly in cognitive intervention programmes for very young children would maximize the chances of providing *continuity of experience*, which, as previously noted, is critical for enhancing the probability of long-term gains.

Intervention at the microsystem level

Microsystem intervention may be viewed at two levels.

At the *family level*, the available evidence continually stresses the detrimental impact on development of a high level of family discord. Thus, one obvious approach is to reduce discord before it can lead to the development of behavioural problems in children. At the very least, a good relationship of the child either with one of the biological parents or with a surrogate parent should be promoted as a means of buffering the effects of family discord (5).

Particularly where there is evidence of biological risk for the young child, it is crucial that parents be trained to be sensitive and responsive to the child's signals. One suggested approach is to reinforce parent behaviour in this direction (185), a strategy that has the virtues not only of increasing the probability of the parents' repeating such behaviour but also of helping to develop in them a sense of their own competence.

Although it may run counter to the culture in many societies, we should try to persuade parents of the detrimental effects of physical punishment, particularly when it is used to deal with school failure or behaviour problems. Teaching parents the relevance of supporting their children's learning activities (173), promoting the use of positive feedback, and utilizing the parent as a valued role model are valid alternatives to punishment (209).

We need to work also with older sibs who are rearing younger brothers and sisters, training them to be more effective, sensitive, and stimulating caretakers (93, 172). Aarons, Hawes, & Gayton's text (286) may be particularly useful in such training.

At the second level, that of the *child*, much of the evidence supporting the general proposition that the environment is relevant to the development of competence is based on the results of provision of some type of supplementary stimulation to children who would not normally have received such stimulation. Perhaps the most clear-cut results involve early psychosocial interventions with young children at risk for mild mental retardation, in which clear gains in cognitive functioning have been reported (213, 287–291).

Although early intervention projects have been shown to have a definite impact on young children's cognitive development, concern has been expressed about the duration of their effects. A recent monograph by Lazar & Darlington (292), who followed up subjects from 12 early intervention projects through adolescence, showed that children who were exposed to psychosocial intervention in the preschool years were more likely to meet later academic requirements and less likely to be held back or assigned to special education classes than were children who did not receive such care. Moreover, the former were found to have greater self-esteem, particularly in terms of academic skills. Generalizability of the gains was evidenced by the fact that mothers of the children who had been in early intervention programmes had higher occupational aspirations for their children over time than did mothers of controls. These findings further support the utilization of early psychosocial intervention as a tool for developing cognitive competence in young children.

Intervention efforts are not restricted to the cognitive sphere. Shure & Spivack (253) have reported that training young children in interpersonal problem-solving and sensitivity to the feelings and needs of other children produces significant gains in competence in interpersonal relations that are maintained for several years.

Two factors must be stressed in any type of psychosocial intervention at the microsystem level.

First, a number of observers have stressed the necessity of making children realistically aware of when they can have an effect on their environment (167, 293–295). Abramson, Seligman, & Teasdale (296) have made a useful distinction between conditions in which a person's actions can help control the outcome and those in which, realistically, they can have no effect. It may be critical, in the latter situation, to help children recognize when this is the case and encourage them to develop alternative goals rather than blame themselves for an undesirable outcome.

In the former situation children should be helped to identify in what specific ways their actions can affect the outcome, and then to act according to what will achieve the desired result. Fowler & Peterson (297) have illustrated how this might be done in terms of children's school achievement.

Second, given the fact of covariance, psychological interventions should not be undertaken in isolation; ideally, they should be combined with a basic service approach (115) involving improved sanitation, better family and child health care, and the production and storage of better-quality food. What this means in practice is that, for maximum input, one should work simultaneously at all levels of the system. An excellent example of this systemwide focus is provided by a psychosocial intervention model developed by MacPhee, Ramey, & Yeates (298), as summarized below:

Steps in a psychosocial intervention model

1. Focus on family social climate and social support before intervention, to reduce stress on the family. Use available community resources to strengthen family functioning.
2. With support networks in place, involve parents as teachers of their children.[2]
   A. Emphasize contingent verbal responses by both parents and sibs.
   B. Emphasize mutual participation in intellectual activities.
   C. Foster a warm relationship between parent and child and show parents how to have fun with their children.
   D. Develop disciplinary techniques that stress reasoning, consistency, and behaviour control.
3. Develop buffering systems to reduce the impact of undesirable aspects of the physical environment.
   A. Develop 'stimulus shelters' for children.
   B. Stress organization of the home environment.
   C. Develop community resources in terms of availability of educational material for children.
4. Be sensitive to age changes and individual differences in children in terms of responsivity to the above.
5. Promote cumulative experiences over time to build on early gains.

Training of personnel

Given the tremendous number of children in need of services and the relatively few trained specialists in child development (299), it seems clear that one-to-one individual therapy is a luxury we cannot afford (277). Perhaps the best way to make maximal use of scarce resources is through Cavalli-Sforza and co-workers' (153) cultural change model, in which a small number of transmitters (specialists) train a large number of respondents (medical officers, teachers), who in turn become transmitters, working with even larger numbers of respondents (children). Several opportunities for such training have been suggested in the literature.

Professionals: physicians and teachers

Particularly in developing countries, the first person contacted for children's behavioural or cognitive problems is often the general medical officer in the community. These professionals have rarely received more than superficial training in the diagnosis and treatment of such problems (299). As a result, parents are all too frequently told that their children 'will grow out of it'. Ideally, child-development specialists should be given the opportunity to teach general medical professionals to identify children's cognitive and behavioural problems reliably, to suggest appropriate treatment, and, when such treatment is beyond the medical professionals' own competence, to make a suitable referral. Whitt & Casey (300) supply an example of how physicians can function in this manner.

In addition to primary-care physicians, another obvious professional resource is teachers. The relevant literature suggests a variety of ways in which teachers can become involved in the diagnosis and remediation of cognitive, motivational, and interpersonal behaviour problems of children *if they are given sufficient training* (256).

Health-care workers

Because of the scarcity of trained personnel, more use of paraprofessional personnel as diagnostic and intervention agents has been stressed (15, 197, 267, 301, 302). Paraprofessional health-care workers could, for example, be employed in the initial screening of children to determine their risk status (156), be involved in early intervention through work with parents to promote cognitive competence (282), act as parent surrogates in cases of loss of parents (193), or work with mothers to develop mutual self-help and self-support groups (132).

The use of health-care workers would seem to have a number of advantages besides the obvious one of increasing the personnel base. Health-care workers who are indigenous to a village or region are likely to be sensitive to relevant family and social values, and hence may be more successful in involving parents in the intervention process than outside specialists would be. Moreover, as a part of the community they are able to follow the children's progress and thus provide the continuity necessary to maximize the impact of the initial interventions (303). Gray & Ruttle (304) have described an excellent example of a cognitive stimulation programme involving indigenous paraprofessionals.

A point that should be stressed with regard to the training of health-care workers is that, given the many factors that determine a child's competence, a *multidisciplinary* training approach should be taken rather than one that focuses narrowly on medical, nutritional, or environmental aspects (115).

Conclusion

I have attempted in this review to show not only the importance of the environment in the development of competence in children but also how the environment works and how knowledge of it can be used to develop intervention strategies. Two areas that seem critical for future research are: (1) identification of the individual parameters that mediate the organism's response to its environment, and (2) development of an understanding of why, in terms of major social stress, some families cope well while others 'go under'. Identification of these individual and family factors would allow us to develop even more effective intervention strategies than those we now employ.

Our ultimate goal must be to utilize our knowledge to devise comprehensive programmes for developing maximal competence in children across a wide range of dimensions. We must realize that our initial gains may not be as dramatic as we should like them to be. Moreover, our interventions may reach only a fraction of the children who need them. An appropriate analogy may be the situation of a child learning to walk: the initial gains are limited, but with increasing coordination and practice, the child does learn to walk. Similarly, our initial gains in helping children to develop competence in facing their changing lives may be small; but with practice in integrating approaches from different disciplines, we will, like the young child, eventually succeed in moving forward confidently and effectively.

Notes

1. For example, moral development and moral judgments fall under cognitive competencies, but these are likely to be highly culturally loaded and therefore less generalizable. Hence, although evidence is available indicating the relevance of parental practices to moral development (22), I shall not be utilizing this aspect of competence in my discussion of the relevance of environment.

2. The characteristics of 'effective teachers' defined in 2 A–D obviously are most salient for an urbanized, Western culture. A different set of parameters may be necessary for different cultures based on different macroenvironmental demand characteristics (76). This outline is thus better viewed as a *process model* rather than a prescription of exactly what to do.

References

1. Crook, T., Raskin, A., & Eliot, P. Parent child relationship and adult depression. *Child Development,* **31**, 785–91 (1974).
2. McCord, J. Some child rearing antecedents of criminal behaviour in adult men. *Journal of Personality and Social Psychology,* **38**, 1377–86 (1979).
3. Robins, L., West, P., & Herjanic, B. Arrest and delinquency in two generations. *Journal of Child Psychology and Psychiatry,* **16**, 125–40 (1975).
4. Siegelman, E., Block, J., Block, J., & Vanderlippe, A. Antecedents of optimal psychological adjustment. *Child Development,* **35**, 283–89 (1970).

5. Rutter, M. Maternal deprivation: 1972–1978. New findings, new concepts, new approaches. *Child Development*, **58**, 283–305 (1979).

6. Skeels, H. Adult status of children with contrasting early life experiences. *Monographs of the Society for Research in Child Development*, **31** (105) (1966).

7. Farrington, D. The family background or aggressive youths. In L. Hersov, M. Berger, & D. Shaffer (Eds.), *Aggression and antisocial behaviour in childhood and adolescence*. Oxford, Pergamon Press, 1978.

8. Hobbs, N. *The troubled and troubling child*. San Francisco, Jossey-Bass, 1982.

9. Lefkowitz, M., Eron, L., Walder, L., & Huesman, L. *Growing up to be violent*. New York, Permagon Press, 1977.

10. Loeber, R., & Dishion, T. Early predictors of male delinquency. *Psychological Bulletin*, **94**, 68–99 (1983).

11. Rutter, M., Yule, W., Berger, M., Yule, B., Morton, J., & Bagley, C. Children of West Indian immigrants. Rates of behaviour deviance and psychiatric disorder. *Journal of Child Psychology and Psychiatry*, **15**, 241–62 (1974).

12. Gold, M. Vocational training. In J. Wortis (Ed.), *Mental retardation and developmental disabilities*. Vol. 7. New York, Brunner/Mazel, 1975.

13. Kirschenbaum, D. Social competence, intervention and evaluation in the inner city. *Journal of Clinical and Consulting Psychology*, **47**, 778–80 (1979).

14. Edgerton, R. Another look at cultural and mental retardation. In M. Begab, H. Haywood, & H. Garber (Eds.), *Psychosocial influences on retarded performance*. Vol. 1. Baltimore, MD, University Park Press, 1981.

15. Lin, T. Mental health in the third world. *Journal of Nervous and Mental Disease*, **171**, 71–78 (1983).

16. Anderson, S., & Messick, S. Social competence in young children. *Developmental Psychology*, **10**, 282–93 (1974).

17. Connolly, K., & Bruner, J. Competence: Its nature and nurture. In K. Connolly & J. Bruner (Eds.), *The growth of competence*. New York, Academic Press, 1974.

18. Diaz-Guerrero, R. The development of coping style. *Human Development*, **27**, 320–31 (1979).

19. White, R. Competence as an aspect of personal growth. In M. Kent & J. Rolf (Eds.), *Primary prevention of psychopathology*. Vol. 3. Hanover, NH, University Press of New England, 1979.

20. Laosa, L. Social competence in childhood. In M. Kent & J. Rolf (Eds.), *Primary prevention of psychopathology*. Vol. 3. Hanover, NH, University Press of New England, 1979.

21. Waters, E., & Sroufe, A. Social competence as a developmental construct. *Developmental Review*, **3**, 57–79 (1983).

22. Leahy, R. Parental practices and the development of moral judgment and self image disparity during adolescence. *Developmental Psychology*, **17**, 580–94 (1981).

23. Bloom, B. *Stability and change in human characteristics*. New York, Wiley, 1964.

24. Wachs, T. D. & Gruen, G. *Early experience and human development*. New York, Plenum, 1982.

25. Block, J., Block, J., & Morrison, A. Parental agreement–disagreement on child rearing orientations and gender related personality correlates in children. *Child Development*, **52**, 965–74 (1981).

26. Howes, C., & Olenick, M. Family and child care influences on toddlers' compliance. *Child Development*, **57**, 202–216 (1986).

27. Marjoribanks, K. Intelligence, social environment and academic achievement, *Journal of Experimental Education*, **47**, 446–52 (1979).

28. Thomas, N., & Berk, L. Effects of school environment on the development of young children's creativity. *Child Development*, **52**, 1153–62 (1981).

29. Emery, R. Interparental conflict and the children of discord and divorce. *Psychological Bulletin*, **92**, 310–30 (1982).

30. Werner, E., & Smith, R. (Eds.) *Vulnerable but invincible*. New York, McGraw-Hill, 1982.

31. Hoffman, J., & Teyber, E. Some relationship between sibling age, spacing and personality. *Merrill Palmer Quarterly*, **25**, 77–80 (1979).

32. Hanson, D., Gottesman, I., & Meehl, P. Genetic theories and the validation of psychiatric diagnosis: Implication for the study of children of schizophrenics. *Journal of Abnormal Psychology*, **6**, 571–88 (1977).

33. Walker, E., & Emory, F. Infants at risk for psychopathology: Offspring of schizophrenic parents. *Child Development*, **54**, 1269–85 (1983).

34. Zubin, J., & Spring, B. Vulnerability – A new view of schizophrenia. *Journal of Abnormal Psychology*, **86**, 103–121 (1977).

35. Crowe, R. An adoption study of antisocial personality. *Archives of General Psychiatry*, **31**, 785–91 (1974).

36. Fallender, C., & Mehrabian, A. Environmental effects of parent–infant interaction. *Genetic Psychology Monographs*, **97**, 3–41 (1978).

37. Murphy, L., & Moriarty, A. *Vulnerability, coping and growth*. New Haven, Yale University Press, 1974.

38. Thomas, A., & Chess, S. Behavioural individuality in childhood. In L. Aronson, E. Tobak, D. Lehrman, & J. Rosenblatt (Eds.), *Development and evolution of behaviour*. San Francisco, Freeman, 1976.

39. Schaeffer, H. Activity level as a constitutional determinant of infantile reaction to deprivation. *Child Development*, **37**, 595–692 (1966).

40. Peters-Martin, P., & Wachs, T. D. A longitudinal study of temperament and its correlates in the first 12 months of life. *Infant Behaviour and Development*, **7**, 288–98 (1984).

41. Wachs, T. D., & Gandour, M. J. Temperament, environment and six-month cognitive intellectual development. *International Journal of Behavioural Development*, **6**, 135–52 (1983).

42. Field, T. Infant arousal, attention and affect during early interaction. In L. Lipsitt (Ed.), *Advances in infant behaviour and development*. Norwood, NJ, Ablex, 1981.

43. Elder, G. *Children of the great depression*. Chicago, University of Chicago Press, 1974.

44. Marjoribanks, K. *Families and their learning environments*. London, Routledge & Kegan Paul, 1979.

45.   Scarr, S., & Weinberg, R. IQ test performance of Black children adopted by white families. *American Psychologist*, **31**, 726–39 (1976).

46.   Bradley, R., & Caldwell, B. The Home Inventory: A validation of the preschool scale for Black children. *Child Development*, **51**, 1140–48 (1981).

47.   Bradley, R., & Caldwell, B. The consistency of the home environment and its relation to child development. *International Journal of Behavioural Development*, **5**, 455–65 (1982).

48.   Clark, E., & Hanisee, J. Intellectual and adaptive performance of Asian children in adoptive American settings. *Developmental Psychology*, **18**, 595–99 (1982).

49.   Clarke, A., & Clarke, A. Early experience: Its limited effect upon later development. In D. Shaffer & J. Dunn (Eds.), *The first year of life*. New York, Wiley, 1979.

50.   Douglas, J. Early hospital admissions and later disturbance of behaviour and learning. *Developmental Medicine and Child Neurology*, **17**, 456–80 (1975).

51.   Early experience and later social behaviour. In D. Shaffer & J. Dunn (Eds.), *The first year of life*. New York, Wiley, 1979.

52.   Tizard, B., & Hodges, J. The effect of early institutional rearing on the development of 8 year old children. *Journal of Child Psychology and Psychiatry*. **19**, 99–118 (1978).

53.   Feuerstein, F., Krasilowsky, D., & Rand, Y. Modifiability during adolescence: Theoretical aspects and empirical data. In E. Anthony & C. Chiland (Eds.), *The child in his family*. Vol. 5. New York, Wiley, 1978.

54.   Bohman, M., & Sigvardsson, S. Long term effects of early institutional care. *Journal of Child Psychology and Psychiatry*, **20**, 111–17 (1979).

55.   Bradley, R., & Caldwell, B. The relation of home environment, cognitive competence and IQ among males and females. *Child Development*, **51**, 1140–48 (1980).

56.   Olson, S., Bates, J., & Bayles, K. Mother–infant interaction and the development of individual differences in children's cognitive competence. *Developmental Psychology*, **20**, 166–79 (1984).

57.   Rutter, M. Family, area and school influences in the genesis of conduct disorders. In L. Hersov, N. Berger, & D. Shaffer (Eds.), *Aggression and anti-social behaviour in childhood and adolescence*. Oxford, Pergamon, 1978.

58.   Klaus, R., & Gray, B. The early training project for disadvantaged children. *Monographs of the Society for Research in Child Development*, **33** (120) (1968).

59.   Bell, R. A reinterpretation of the direction of effects in studies of socialization. *Psychological Review*, **75**, 1163–70 (1980).

60.   Sameroff, A., & Chandler, N. Reproductive risk and the continuum of care taking causality. In F. Horowitz (Ed.), *Review of child development research*. Chicago, University of Chicago Press, 1975.

61.   Bradley, R., Caldwell, B., & Elardo, R. Home environment and cognitive development in the first two years. *Developmental Psychology*, **15**, 246–50 (1979).

62.   Irwin, M., Engle, P., Yarbrough, C., Klein, R., & Townsend, J. The relationship

of prior ability and family characteristics to school attendance and school achievement in rural Guatemala. *Child Development*, **49**, 415–27 (1978).

63. Lester, B. A synergistic process approach to the study of prenatel malnutrition. *International Journal of Behavioural Development*, **2**, 377–93 (1979).

64. Super, C., Clement, J., Vuori, L., Christiansen, N., Mora, J., & Herrera, M. Caretaker behaviour as mediator of nutritional and social interaction in the barrios of Bogota. In T. Field (Ed.), *Culture and early interaction*. Hillsdale, NJ, Erlbaum, 1981.

65. Zeskind, P., & Ramsey, C. Preventing intellectual and interactional sequelae of fetal malnutrition. *Child Development*, **52**, 213–18 (1981).

66. DeVries, M. Temperament and infant mortality among the Masai of East Africa. *American Journal of Psychiatry*, **171**, 1189–97 (1987).

67. Bronfenbrenner, U. Toward an experimental ecology of human development. *American Psychologist*, **32**, 513–31 (1977).

68. Wohlwill, J. The concept of experience: S or R. *Human Development*, **16**, 90–107 (1973).

69. Rowe, D., & Plomin, R. The importance of non-shared environmental influences in behavioural development. *Developmental Psychology*, **17**, 517–31 (1981).

70. Wohlwill, J. Physical and social environments as factors in development. In D. Magnusson & V. Allen (Eds.), *Human development: An interactional perspective*. New York, Academic Press, 1983.

71. Berry, J. Nomadic style and cognitive style. In H. McGurk (Ed.), *Ecological factors in human development*. Amsterdam, North Holland, 1977.

72. Cotterell, J. Work and community influences on the quality of child rearing. *Child Development*, **57**, 362–74 (1986).

73. Kagan, S., & Ender, P. Maternal response to success and failure of Anglo American, Mexican American and Mexican children. Child Development, **31**, 319–32 (1972).

74. Marvin, R., Van Devender, T., Iwanaga, M., LeVine, S., & LeVine, R. Infant caregiver attachment among the Hausa of Nigeria. In H. McGurk (Ed.), *Ecological factors in human development*. Amsterdam, North Holland, 1977.

75. McSwain, R. Care and conflict in infant development. *Infant Behaviour and Development*, **200**, 270–78 (1978).

76. Ogbu, J. Origins of human competence: A cultural-ecological perspective. *Child Development*, **52**, 413–29 (1981).

77. Shouval, R., Venoki, S., Bronfenbrenner, U., Devereaux, E., & Kieley, E. Anomalous reactions to social pressure of Israeli and Soviet children raised in families versus collective settings. *Journal of Personality and Social Psychology*, **32**, 477–89 (1975).

78. Witkin, H., & Berry, J. Psychological differentiation in cross-cultural perspective. *Journal of Cross-cultural Psychology*, **6**, 4–87 (1975).

79. Valsiner, J. The father's role in the social network of a Soviet child. In M. Lamb (Ed.), *The role of the father in child development* (2nd ed.). New York, Wiley, 1981.

80. McClelland, D. Child rearing versus ideology and social structure. In R. Munroe, R. Munroe, & B. Whiting (Eds.), *Handbook of cross-cultural human development.* New York, Garland, 1981.

81. Montare, A., & Boone, S. Aggression and paternal absence: Racial and ethnic differences among inner-city boys. *Journal of Genetic Psychology,* **137**, 223–32 (1980).

82. Knight, G., Kagan, S., & Buriel, R. Perceived parental practices and prosocial development. *Journal of Genetic Psychology,* **141**, 57–61 (1982)

83. Buriel, R. The relation of Anglo and Mexican American children's locus of control beliefs to parents' and children's socialization practices. *Child Development,* **52**, 104–113 (1981).

84. Rutter, M., & Quinton, D. Psychiatric disorders; Ecological factors and concepts of causation. In H. McGurk (Ed.), *Ecological factors in human development.* Amsterdam, North Holland, 1977.

85. Earls, F., & Richman, N. Behaviour problems in preschool children of West Indian born parents. *Journal of Child Psychology and Psychiatry,* **21**, 107–117 (1980).

86. Taylor, L. Family environment, language and intelligence. *Canadian Journal of Behavioural Sciences,* **11**, 1–10 (1979).

87. Udwin, O., & Schmukler, D. The influence of sociocultural, economic and home background factors on children's ability to engage in imaginative play. *Developmental Psychology,* **17**, 66–72 (1981).

88. Coelho, G., & Stein, J. Coping with rapid change: New stress in human settlements. In E. Anthony & C. Chiland (Eds.), *The child in his family.* Vol. 6. New York, Wiley, 1980.

89. Lieh-Mak, F. Boat children: The implication of high density living. In E. Anthony & C. Chiland (Eds.), *The child in his family.* Vol. 6. New York, Wiley, 1980.

90. Hunt, J. McV. *Specificity in early development and experience.* O'Neil invited lecture. Myer Children's Rehabilitation Institute, University of Nebraska Medical Centre, Omaha, NB, 1977.

91. Hunt, J. McV. Psychological development: Early experience. *Annual Review of Psychology,* **30**, 103–44 (1979).

92. Wachs, T. D. The use and abuse of environment in behaviour genetic research. *Child Development,* **54**, 396–407 (1983).

93. Wachs, T. D. Proximal experience and early cognitive intellectual development: The social environment. In A. Gottfried (Ed.), *Home environment and early development.* New York, Academic Press, 1985.

94. Haggard, E., & Van DerLippe, A. Isolated families in the mountains of Norway. In E. Anthony & C. Koupernik (Eds.), *The child in his family.* Vol. 1. New York, Wiley, 1970.

95. Hollos, M., & Cowan, P. Social isolation and cognitive development. *Child Development,* **44**, 630–41 (1973).

96. Nerlove, S., & Snipper, A. Cognitive consequences of cultural opportunities. In R. Munroe, R. Munroe, & B. Whiting (Eds.), *Handbook of cross-cultural human development.* New York, Garland, 1981.

97. Soar, R. Teaching behaviours and measures of pupil growth. *International Review of Education*, **18**, 508–28 (1972).

98. Hatano, G., Mizake, K., & Tajima, N. Mother's behaviour in an unstructured situation and child's acquisition of number conversation. *Child Development*, **51**, 379–85 (1980).

99. Iverson, B., & Walberg, H. Home environment and school learning: A quantitative synthesis. *Journal of Experimental Education*, **50**, 144–51 (1982).

100. Kelleghan, T. Relationships between home environment and scholastic behaviour in a disadvantaged population. *Journal of Educational Psychology*, **69**, 754–60 (1977).

101. Kirk, L. Maternal and subcultural correlates of cognitive growth rate. In P. Dasen (Ed.), *Piagetian psychology: Cross cultural contributions*. New York, Halstead, 1977.

102. Shinn, M. Father absence and children's cognitive development. *Psychological Bulletin*, **85**, 295–324 (1978).

103. Wachs, T. D., & Chan, A. Specificity of environmental action as seen in physical and social environmental correlates of three aspects of twelve months infants' communication performance. *Child Development*. **57**, 1464–75 (1986).

104. Folner, R., Stolborg, A., & Cowon, E. Crisis events and school mental health referral patterns of young children. *Journal of Clinical and Consulting Psychology*, **43**, 305–310 (1975).

105. Rutter, M. Stress coping and development: Some issues and some questions. *Journal of Child Psychology and Psychiatry*, **22**, 323–56 (1981).

106. Fritsch, T., & Burkhead, J. Behavioural reaction of children to parental absence due to imprisonment. *Family Relations*, **30**, 83–88 (1981).

107. Block, J. *Lives through time*. Berkeley, CA, Bancroft, 1971.

108. Goldstein, M. Family factors associated with schizophrenia and anorexia nervosa. *Journal of Youth and Adolescence*, **10**, 385 (1981).

109. Newcomb, M., Huba, G., & Bentler, P. Mother's influence on the drug use of their children. *Developmental Psychology*, **19**, 714–26 (1983).

110. Brozek, J. Nutrition, malnutrition and behaviour. *Annual Review of Psychology*, **29**, 157–77 (1978).

111. Gabr, M. Malnutrition during pregnancy and lactation. *World Review of Nutrition and Diet*, **36**, 90–99 (1981).

112. Herrera, M., Christiansen, N., Ortiz, N., Clement, J., Vuori, L. Parades, D., Wagner, G., & Weber, D. Effects of nutritional supplementation and early education on physical and cognitive development. In R. Turner & H. Reese (Eds.), *Lifespan developmental psychology*. New York, Academic Press, 1980.

113. Lloyd-Still, J. Clinical studies on the effects of malnutrition during infancy on subsequent physical and intellectual development. In J. Lloyd-Still (Ed.), *Malnutrition and intellectual development*. Littleton, MA, Publishing Sciences Group, 1976.

114. Riciutti, H. Adverse social and biological influences on early development. In H. McGurk (Ed.), *Ecological factors in human development*. Amsterdam, North Holland, 1977.

96   *Theodore D. Wachs*

115. Werner, E. *Cross-cultural child development.* Monterey, CA, Brooks-Cole, 1979.
116. Craviotto, J., & Delicardi, E. Environmental correlates of severe clinical malnutrition and language development in survivors from kwashiorkor or marasmus. In Pan American Health Organization, *Nutrition: The nervous system and behaviour* (Publication no. 251). Washington, DC, PAHO, 1972.
117. Joffe, J. Approaches to prevention of adverse developmental consequences of genetic and prenatal factors. In L. Bond & J. Joffe (Eds.), *Facilitating infant and early childhood development.* Hanover, NH, University Press of New England, 1982.
118. Kopp, C., & Parmelee, A. Prenatal and perinatal influences on infant behaviour. In J. Osofsky (Ed.), *Handbook of infant development.* New York, Wiley, 1979.
119. Tarjan, G. The prevention of psycho-social retardation. In E. Anthony & C. Chiland (Eds.), *The child in his family.* Vol. 6. New York, Wiley, 1980.
120. Haywood, H., & Wachs, T. D. Intelligence, cognition and individual differences. In M. Begab, H. Haywood, & H. Garber (Eds.), *Psychosocial influences in retarded performance.* Vol. 1. Baltimore, MD, University Park Press, 1981.
121. Sameroff, A., & Seifer, R. Family risk and child competence. *Child Development,* **54**, 1254–68 (1983).
122. Sameroff, A., & McDonough, S. The role of motor activity in human cognitive and social development. In E. Pollitt & P. Amante (Eds.), *Early intake and activity.* New York, Liss, 1984.
123. Scarr, S. Constructing psychology: Making facts and fables for our times. *American Psychologist,* **40**, 499–512 (1985).
124. Sigman, M. Plasticity in development: Implications for intervention. In L. Bond & J. Joffe (Eds.), *Facilitating infant and early childhood development.* Hanover, NH, University Press of New England, 1982.
125. Sharpe, D., Cole, M., & Laver, C. Education and cognitive development. *Monographs of the Society for Research in Child Development,* **44** (178) (1979).
126. Graham, P. Environmental influences on psychosocial development. *International Journal of Mental Health,* **6** (3), 7–31 (1977).
127. Lambo, T. The vulnerable African child. In E. Anthony & C. Koupernik (Eds.), *The child in his family.* Vol. 3. New York, Wiley, 1974.
128. Leng, Y., & Ong, S. Malaysian child psychiatry practices. *Australian and New Zealand Journal of Psychiatry,* **16**, 61–66 (1982).
129. Sanda, A. The Nigerian family in transition. In E. Anthony & C. Chiland (Eds.), *The child in his family.* Vol. 7. New York, Wiley, 1982.
130. Asuni, T. Socio-psychological aspects of the vulnerable child: Risk and mastery: Children of the modern elite in Nigeria. In E. Anthony & C. Koupernik (Eds.), *The child in his family.* Vol. 3. New York, Wiley, 1974.
131. Thanaphum, S. Understanding and ensuring normal adolescent development in Thailand. In E. Anthony & C. Chiland (Eds.), *The child in his family.* Vol. 6. New York, Wiley, 1980.
132. Chaplan, G. Family support systems in a changing world. In E. Anthony & C. Chiland (Eds.), *The child in his family.* Vol. 5. New York, Wiley, 1978.
133. Morice, R. Change in the aboriginal adolescent. In E. Anthony & C. Chiland (Eds.), *The child in his family.* Vol. 6. New York, Wiley, 1980.

134. Weisner, J. Cities, stress and children. In R. Munroe, R. Munroe, & R. Whiting (Eds.), *Handbook of cross-cultural human development.* New York, Garland, 1981.

135. Davidson, G. Child rearing as a response to traditional aboriginal and modern Western value systems. In E. Anthony & C. Chiland (Eds.), *The child in his family.* Vol. 6. New York, Wiley, 1980.

136. Milgram, R., & Milgram, N. The effects of the Yom Kippur war on anxiety level in Israeli children. *Journal of Psychology,* **94,** 107–113 (1976).

137. Garmezy, N. Stressors of childhood. In N. Garmezy & M. Rutter (Eds.), *Stress, coping and development in children.* New York, McGraw-Hill, 1983.

138. Klingman, A., & Wiesner, E. The relationship of proximity to tension areas and size of settlement to fear level of Israeli children. *Journal of Behaviour Therapy and Experimental Psychiatry,* **13,** 321–23 (1982).

139. Levy-Shiff, R. The effects of father absence on young children in mother headed families. *Child Development,* **53,** 1400–1405 (1982).

140. McWhirter, L., & Trew, K. Children in Northern Ireland: A lost generation? In E. Anthony & C. Chiland (Eds.), *The child in his family.* Vol. 7. New York, Wiley, 1982.

141. Fields, R. Child terror victims and adult terrorists. *Journal of Psychohistory,* **7,** 71–75 (1979).

142. Wohlwill, J., & Heft, H. Environments fit for the developing child. In H. McGurk (Ed.), *Ecological factors in human development.* Amsterdam, North Holland, 1977.

143. Stevenson, H., Parke, T., Wilkinson, A., Bonnevaux, B., & Gonzalez, M. Schooling, environment and cognitive development: A cross-cultural study. *Monographs of the Society for Research in Child Development,* **43** (175) (1978).

144. Rogoff, B. Schooling and the development of cognitive skills. In H. Triandis & A. Heron (Eds.), *Handbook of cross-cultural psychology.* Boston, Allyn & Bacon, 1981.

145. Rutter, M. School effects on pupils progress. Research findings and policy implications. *Child Development,* **54,** 1–29 (1983).

146. Busse, T., Ree, M., Gutride, M., Alexander, T., & Powell, L. Environmentally enriched classrooms and the cognitive and perceptual development of Negro preschool children. *Journal of Educational Psychology,* **63,** 15–21 (1982).

147. Cochran, N., & Brossard, J. Child development and personal-social networks. *Child Development,* **50,** 601–616 (1979).

148. Bee, H., Barnard, K., Eyres, S., Gray, C., Hammond, M., Spietz, A., Snyder, C., & Clark, B. Prediction of IQ and language skill from perinatal status, child performance, family characteristics and mother infant interaction. *Child Development,* **53,** 1134–56 (1982).

149. Pascoe, J., Loda, F., Jeffries, V., & Earp, J. The association between mothers' social support and provision of stimulation to their children. *Journal of Developmental and Behavioural Pediatrics,* **2,** 15–19 (1981).

150. Weinraub, M., & Wolf, B. Effects of stress and social supports on mother-child interactions in single and two parent families. *Child Development,* **54,** 1297–1311 (1983).

98   *Theodore D. Wachs*

151. Crockenberg, S., & McCluskey, K. Change in maternal behaviour during the baby's first year of life. *Child Development,* **57**, 746–53 (1986).
152. Hess, R. Social competence and the educational process. In K. Connolly & J. Bruner (Eds.), *The growth of competence.* New York, Academic Press, 1974.
153. Cavalli-Sforza, L., Feldman, M., Chen, K., & Dornbusch, S. Theory and observation in cultural transmission. *Science,* **218**, 19–27 (1982).
154. Watts, D. Discontinuity between home and school as a hazard in child development. In E. Anthony & C. Koupernik (Eds.), *The child in his family.* Vol. 4. New York, Wiley, 1978.
155. Cederblad, N. A child psychiatric study on Sudanese Arab children. *Acta Psychiatrica Scandinavica,* Suppl. 200 (1968).
156. Graham, P., & Canavan, K. The mental health of children in developing countries. In E. Anthony & C. Chiland (Eds.), *The child in his family.* Vol. 7. New York, Wiley, 1982.
157. Marjoribanks, K. An Adlerian typology of school learning environments and children's feeling of inferiority. *Psychological Reports,* **47**, 787–94 (1980).
158. Gump, P. School environments. In I. Altman & J. Wohlwill (Eds.), *Children in the environment.* New York, Plenum, 1978.
159. Arlin, M., & Whitley, T. Perception of self-managed learning opportunities and academic locus of control. *Journal of Educational Psychology,* **70**, 988–92 (1978).
160. Rosen, C. The impact of an open campus program upon high school students' sense of control over their environment. *Psychology in the School,* **14**, 216–19 (1977).
161. Winefield, A., & Fay, P. Effects of an institutional environment on responses to uncontrollable outcomes. *Motivation and Emotion,* **6**, 103–112 (1982).
162. Dean, A., & Lin, N. The stress buffering role of social support. *Journal of Nervous and Mental Disease,* **165**, 403–417 (1977).
163. Gottfried, A. Home environment and early mental development: Integration, metaanalysis and conclusions. In A. Gottfried (Ed.), *Home environment and early mental development.* New York, Academic Press, 1984.
164. Crawley, S., & Spiker, D. Mother child interaction involving two-year-olds with Down's syndrome. *Child Development,* **54**, 1312–23 (1983).
165. Gaiter, J., Morgan, G., Jennings, K., Harmon, R., & Yarrow, L. Variety of cognitively oriented caregiver activities: Relationship to cognitive and motivational functioning at 1 and $3\frac{1}{2}$ years of age. *Journal of Genetic Psychology,* **141**, 49–56 (1982).
166. Poresky, R., & Henderson, M. Infants' mental and motor development: Effects of home environment, maternal attitudes, marital adjustment and socioeconomic status. *Perceptual and Motor Skills,* **64**, 695–702 (1982).
167. Ramey, C., & McPhee, D. Developmental retardation among the poor: A systems theory perspective on risk and prevention. In D. Farran & J. McKinney (Eds.), *Risk in intellectual and psychosocial development.* New York, Academic Press. In press.
168. Van Doorninck, W., Caldwell, B., Wright, C., & Frankenburg, W. Relationship between 12 month home stimulation and school achievement. *Child Development,* **52**, 1080–83 (1981).

169. Smith, I., & Hagen, V. Relationship between the home environment and sensorimotor development of Down's syndrome and non-retarded infants. *American Journal of Mental Deficiency.* **89**, 124–32 (1984).

170. Goldberg, S. Parent–infant bonding: Another look. *Child Development,* **54**, 1355–82 (1983).

171. Wiberg, B., & DeChateau, P. Long-term effects on mother–infant behaviour of extra contact during the first hour post-partum. In E. Anthony & C. Chiland (Eds.), *The child in his family.* Vol. 7. New York, Wiley, 1982.

172. Norman-Jackson, J. Family interaction, language development and primary reading achievement of Black children in families of low income. *Child Development,* **53**, 349–58 (1982).

173. Parkinson, C., Wallis, S., Prince, J., & Harvey, D. Rating the home environment of school age children: A comparison with general cognitive index and school progress. *Journal of Child Psychology and Psychiatry,* **23**, 329–33 (1982).

174. Seginer, R. Parents' educational expectations and children's academic achievement: A literature review. *Merrill–Palmer Quarterly,* **29**, 1–23 (1983).

175. Hanson, R. Consistency and stability of home environmental measures related to IQ. *Child Development,* **46**, 470–80 (1975).

176. Kent, N., & Davis, R. Discipline in the home and intellectual development. *British Journal of Medical Psychology,* **30**, 27–33 (1957).

177. McCall, R., Appelbaum, M., & Hogarty, P. Developmental change in mental performance. *Monographs of the Society for Research in Child Development,* **38** (150) (1973).

178. Witkin, H. Socialization, culture and ecology in the development of group and sex differences in cognitive style. *Human Development,* **22**, 358–72 (1979).

179. Rankin, R., Gaiter, A., & Heiry, T. Cultural modification of effect of family size on intelligence. *Psychological Reports,* **45**, 391–97 (1979).

180. Zajonc, R. Family configuration and intelligence. *Science,* **192**, 227–36 (1976).

181. Zajonc, R. Validating the confluence model. *Psychological Bulletin,* **93**, 457–80 (1983).

182. Walberg, H., & Marjoribanks, K. Family environment and cognitive development: 12 analytic models. *Review of Educational Research,* **46**, 527–51 (1976).

183. Brackbill, Y., & Nichols, P. A test of the confluence model of intellectual development. *Development Psychology,* **18**, 192–98 (1982).

184. Ide, J., Parkerson, J., Haertal, G., & Walberg, H. Peer group influences on educational outcomes. *Journal of Educational Psychology,* **73**, 473–94 (1981).

185. Belsky, J., Goode, M., & Most, R. Maternal stimulation and infant exploratory competence. *Child Development,* **51**, 1163–70 (1980).

186. Jennings, K., Harmon, R., Morgan, G., Gaiter, J., & Yarrow, L. Exploratory play as an index of mastery motivation. Relationship to persistence, cognitive functioning and environmental measures. *Developmental Psychology,* **15**, 366–74 (1979).

187. Power, T., & Chapieski, L. Child rearing and impulse control in toddlers. *Developmental Psychology,* **22**, 271–75 (1986).

188. Yarrow, L., Morgan, J., Jennings, K., Harmon, R., & Gaiter, J. *Infant Behaviour and Development,* **5,** 131–41 (1982).

189. Yarrow, L., MacTurk, R., Vietze, P., McCarthy, M., Klein, R., & McQuiston, S. The developmental course of parental stimulation and its relation to mastery motivation during infancy. *Developmental Psychology,* **20,** 492–503 (1987).

190. Radin, N. Primary caregiving and role sharing fathers. In M. Lamb (Ed.), *Nontraditional families,* Hillsdale, NJ, Erlbaum, 1982.

191. Sagi, A. Antecedents and consequence of various degrees of paternal involvement in child rearing. In M. Lamb (Ed.), *Nontraditional families.* Hillsdale, NJ, Erlbaum, 1982.

192. Bradley, R. Preschool home environment and classroom behaviour. *Journal of Experimental Education,* **49,** 196–99 (1982).

193. Fry, P., & Grover, S. The relationship between father absence and children's social problem solving competencies. *Journal of Applied Developmental Psychology,* **3,** 105–120 (1982).

194. Bacon, M., Child, I., & Barry, H. A cross-cultural study of the correlates of crime. *Journal of Abnormal and Social Psychology,* **66,** 291–300 (1963).

195. Ember, C. A cross-cultural perspective on sex differences. In R. Munroe, R. Munroe, & B. Whiting (Eds.), *Handbook of cross-cultural human development.* New York, Garland, 1981.

196. Katz, M., & Konner, M. The role of the father: An anthropological perspective. In M. Lamb (Ed.), *The role of the father in child development* (2nd ed.). New York, Wiley, 1981.

197. Minde, K. Children in Uganda: Rates of behavioural deviation and psychiatric disorder in various school and clinic populations. *Journal of Child Psychology and Psychiatry,* **18,** 23–37 (1977).

198. Klein, M., & Shulman, S. Behaviour problems of children in relation to parental instrumentality–expressivity and marital adjustment. *Psychological Reports,* **47,** 11–14 (1980).

199. Emery, R., Weintrub, S., & Neale, J. Effects of marital discord on the school behaviour of children of schizophrenic, affectively disordered and normal parents. *Journal of Abnormal Child Psychology,* **10,** 215–28 (1982).

200. Nihara, K., Mink, I., & Meyers, C. Relationship between home environment and school adjustment of TMR children. *American Journal of Mental Deficiency,* **86,** 8–15 (1981).

201. Forman, S., & Forman, B. Family environment and its relation to adolescent personality factors. *Journal of Personality Assessment,* **45,** 163–67 (1981).

202. Jacob, T. Family interaction in disturbed and normal families. *Psychological Bulletin,* **82,** 33–65 (1975).

203. Wynne, L. Current concepts about schizophrenics and family relationships. *Journal of Nervous and Mental Disease,* **169,** 82–89 (1981).

204. Fisher, L., & Jones, J. Child competence and psychiatric risk. *Journal of Nervous and Mental Disease,* **168,** 332–37 (1980).

205. Main, M., & George, C. Responses of abused and disadvantaged toddlers to distress in agemates. *Developmental Psychology,* **21,** 707–712 (1985).

206. Zarb, J. Correlates of recidivism and social adjustment among training school delinquents. *Canadian Journal of Behavioural Science,* **10**, 317–28 (1978).

207. Barling, J. Maternal antecendents of children's multidimensional locus of control beliefs. *Journal of Genetic Psychology,* **140**, 155–56 (1982).

208. Cole, R., Baldwin, A., Baldwin, C., & Fisher, L. Family interaction in free play and children's social competence. In A. Baldwin, R. Cole, & C. Baldwin, Parental pathology, family interaction and the competence of the child in school. *Monographs of the Society for Research in Child Development,* **47** (197) (1982).

209. Simeonsson, R. Social competence. In J. Wortis, *Mental retardation and developmental disabilities.* Vol. 10. New York, Brunner/Mazel, 1978.

210. Piper, M., & Ramsay, M. Effect of early home environment on the mental development of Down's syndrome infants. *American Journal of Mental Deficiency,* **85**, 39–44 (1980).

211. Shipe, D., & Shotwell, A. Effects of out of home care on mongoloid children. *American Journal of Mental Deficiency,* **69**, 649–52 (1965).

212. Stedman, D., & Eichorn, D. A comparison of the growth and development of institutionalized and home reared mongoloids during infancy and early childhood. *American Journal of Mental Deficiency,* **69**, 391–401 (1964).

213. Caldwell, B., Bradley, R., & Elardo, R. Early stimulation. In J. Wortis (Ed.), *Mental retardation and developmental disabilities.* Vol. 7. New York, Brunner/Mazel, 1975.

214. Hanson, M. Down's syndrome children: Characteristics and intervention research. In M. Lewis & L. Rosenblum (Eds.), *The uncommon child.* New York, Plenum, 1981.

215. Hayden, A., & Dmitriev, V. The multidisciplinary program for Down's syndrome children at the University of Washington Model Preschool Center. In G. Friedlander, G. Sterritt, & G. Kirk (Eds.), *Exceptional infant.* Vol. 3. New York, Brunner/Mazel, 1975.

216. Anthony, E. The syndrome of the psychologically vulnerable child. In E. Anthony & C. Koupernik (Eds.), *The child in his family.* Vol. 3. New York, Wiley, 1974.

217. Mednick, S., Schulsinger, H., & Schulsinger, F. Schizophrenia in children of schizophrenic mothers. In A. Davids (Ed.), *Child personality and psychopathology.* New York, Wiley, 1975.

218. Schulsinger, F. Biological psychopathology. *Annual Review of Psychology,* **3**, 583–606 (1980).

219. Hutchings, B., & Mednick, S. Registered criminality in the adoptive and biological parents of registered male criminal adoptees. In R. Fieve, D. Rosenthal, & D. Bill (Eds.), *Genetics research in psychiatry.* Baltimore, MD, Johns Hopkins University Press, 1975.

220. Venables, P., Mednick, S., Schulsinger, F., Raman, A., Bell, B., Dalais, C., & Fletcher, R. Screening for risk of mental illness. In G. Serban (Ed.), *Cognitive deficits in the development of mental illness.* New York, Brunner/Mazel, 1978.

221. Anderson, L., Dancis, J., Alpert, M., & Herrman, L. Punishment learning and self-mutilation in Lesch-Nyhan Disease. *Nature,* **265**, 461–63 (1977).

222. Broman, S., Nichols, P., & Kennedy, W. *Preschool IQ: Prenatal and early development correlates*. New York, Wiley, 1975.

223. Willerman, L., Broman, S., & Fiedler, M. Infant development, preschool IQ and social class. *Child Development*, **41**, 69–77 (1979).

224. Beckwith, L., & Cohen, S. Home environment and cognitive competence in preterm children in the first five years. In A. Gottfried (Ed.), *Home environment and early mental development*. New York, Academic Press, 1984.

225. Beckwith, L., Cohen, J., Kopp, C., Parmelee, A., & Marcy, J. Caregiver infant interaction and early cognitive development in pre-term infants. *Child Development*, **47**, 579–87 (1976).

226. Jordon, T., & Spooner, S. Biological and ecological influences on development at 24 and 36 months of age. *Psychological Reports*, **31**, 319–32 (1972).

227. Werner, E., Bierman, J., & French, F. *The children of Kauai: A longitudinal study from the pre-natal period to age 10*. Honolulu, University of Hawaii Press, 1977.

228. Beckwith, L., & Parmelee, A. EEG patterns of pre-term infants, home environment and later IQ. *Child Development*, **57**, 777–89 (1986).

229. Scarr, S., & Williams, M. The effects of early stimulation on low birth weight infants. *Child Development*, **44**, 94–101 (1973).

230. Barnard, K., & Bee, H. The impact of temporally patterned stimulation on the development of pre-term infants. *Child Development*, **54**, 1156–67 (1983).

231. Cornell, E., & Gottfried, A. Intervention with premature infants. *Child Development*, **47**, 32–39 (1976).

232. Katz, V. Auditory stimulation and developmental behaviour of the premature infant. *Nursing Research*, **20**, 196–210 (1971).

233. Powell, L. The effect of extra stimulation and maternal involvement on the development of low birth weight infants and on maternal behaviour. *Child Development*, **45**, 106–113 (1974).

234. Siqueland, E. Biological and experimental determinants of exploration in infancy. In L. Stone, H. Smith, & L. Murphy (Eds.), *The competent infant*. New York, Basic Books, 1973.

235. Solkoff, N., & Matuszak, D. Tactile stimulation and behavioural development among low birth weight infants. *Child Psychiatry and Human Development*, **6**, 33–37 (1975).

236. Solkoff, N., & Sumner, D., Weintraub, D., & Blase, B. Effects of handling on the subsequent development of premature infants. *Developmental Psychology*, **1**, 765–68 (1969).

237. Williams, M., & Scarr, S. Effects of short term intervention on performance in low birth weight disadvantaged infants. *Pediatrics*, **47**, 289–98 (1971).

238. Kahn, J. Acceleration of object permanence with severely and profoundly retarded children. *American Association for the Severely Profoundly Handicapped Review*, **3**, 15–22 (1978).

239. Vogel, W., Kan, K., & Meshorer, E. Effects of environmental enrichment and environmental deprivation on cognitive functioning in institutionalized retardates. *Journal of Consulting Psychology*, **31**, 570–76 (1967).

240. Horner, R. The effect of an environmental enrichment program on the behaviour of institutionalized profoundly retarded children. *Journal of Applied Behavioural Analysis*, **3**, 477–91 (1980).

241. Nihara, K., Mink, I., & Meyers, E. Salient dimensions of home environment relevant to child development. In N. Ellis & N. Bray (Eds.), *International review of research in mental retardation*. Vol. 12. New York, Academic Press, 1984.

242. Zeskind, P., & Ramey, C. Fetal malnutrition: An experimental study of its consequences on infant development in 2 caregiving environments. *Child Development*, **48**, 1155–62 (1978).

243. Bejar, I. Does nutrition cause intelligence? A reanalysis of the Cali experiment. *Intelligence*, **5**, 49–68 (1982).

244. Richardson, S. The relation of severe malnutrition in infancy to the intelligence of school children with differing life histories. *Pediatric Research*, **10**, 57–61 (1976).

245. Winick, M., Meyer, K., & Harris, R. Malnutrition and environmental enrichment by early adoption. *Science*, **190**, 1173–75 (1975).

246. Karnes, M., Teska, J., & Hodgins, A. The effects of four programs of classroom intervention on the intellectual and language development of 4 year old disadvantaged children. *American Journal of Orthopsychiatry*, **40**, 58–76 (1970).

247. Levenstein, P. Cognitive growth in preschoolers through verbal interactions with mothers. *American Journal of Orthopsychiatry*, **40**, 426–32 (1970).

248. Madden, J., Levenstein, P., & Levenstein, P. Longitudinal IQ outcomes of the mother child home program. *Child Development*, **47**, 1015–25 (1976).

249. Karnes, M., Teska, J., Hodgins, A., & Badger, E. Educational intervention of home by mothers of disadvantaged infants. *Child Development*, **41**, 925–35 (1970).

250. Ramey, C., McPhee, D., & Yeates, K. Preventing developmental retardation: A general systems model. In L. Bond & J. Joffe (Eds.), *Facilitating infant and early childhood development*. Hanover, NH, University Press of New England, 1982.

251. Hunt, J., McV. Facilitating the development of social competence and language skills. In L. Bond & J. Joffe (Eds.), *Facilitating infant and early childhood development*. Hanover, NH, University Press of New England, 1982.

252. Oshman, H., & Manosevitz, M. Father absence: Effects of stepfathers upon psychosocial development in males. *Developmental Psychology*, **12**, 479–80 (1976).

253. Shure, M., & Spivack, G. Interpersonal problem solving, thinking and adjustment of the mother-child dyad. In M. Kent & J. Rolf (Eds.), *Primary prevention of psychopathology*. Vol. 3. Hanover, NH, University Press of New England, 1979.

254. Reid, J., & Patterson, G. The modification of aggression and stealing behaviour of boys in the home setting. In E. Ribes-Inesta & A. Bandura (Eds.), *Analysis of delinquency and aggression*. Hillsdale, NJ, Erlbaum, 1976.

255. Marcus, J. Planning of comprehensive preventative care for the vulnerable child population. In E. Anthony, C. Koupernik, & C. Chiland (Eds.), *The child in his family*. Vol. 4. New York, Wiley, 1978.

256. Vaughn, P., Boorse, E., & Jacobi, S. Mental health at the preschool level. In E.

Anthony, C. Koupernik, & C. Chiland (Eds.), *The child in his family.* Vol. 4. New York, Wiley, 1978.

257. Rosenfeld, E., & Barder, L. A compensatory community environment for the culturally disadvantaged child. In E. Anthony, C. Koupernik, & C. Chiland (Eds.), *The child in his family.* Vol. 4. New York, Wiley, 1978.

258. Escalona, S. Intervention programs for children of psychiatric risk. In E. Anthony & C. Koupernik (Eds.), *The child in his family.* Vol. 3. New York, Wiley, 1974.

259. Werner, E., & Smith, R. *Kauai's children come of age.* Honolulu, University of Hawaii Press, 1977.

260. Kopp, C. Individual differences and intervention for infants and young children. *Journal of Pediatric Psychology,* **3**, 145–49 (1978).

261. Segal, J. Utilization of stress and coping research. In N. Garmezy & M. Rutter (Eds.), *Coping and development in children.* New York, McGraw-Hill, 1983.

262. Werner, E. *Child care:*Kith, kin and hired hands. Baltimore, MD, University Park Press, 1984.

263. McCall, R., Gregory, T., & Murray, J. Communicating developmental research results to the general public through television. *Developmental Psychology,* **20**, 45–54 (1984).

264. Roberts, D., & Bachen, C. Mass communication effects. *Annual Review of Psychology,* **32**, 307–356 (1981).

265. Hasan, K. Effect on child mental health of psychosocial change in developing countries. *International Journal of Mental Health,* **6** (3), 49–57 (1977).

266. Brown, J., LaRossa, M., Aylward, G., Davis, D., Rutherford, P., & Bakeman, R. Nursery based intervention with prematurely born babies and their mothers. *Journal of Pediatrics,* **97**, 487–91 (1980).

267. Zigler, E., & Finn, M. A vision of child care in the 1980's. In L. Bond & J. Joffe (Eds.), *Facilitating infant and early childhood development.* Hanover, NH, University Press of New England, 1982.

268. Schiff, M., Duyme, M., Dumaret, A., Stewart, J., Tomkiewicz, S., & Feingold, J. Intellectual status of working class children adopted early in upper middle class families. *Science,* **200**, 1503–1504 (1978).

269. Clark, E., & Hanisee, J. Intellectual and adaptive performance of Asian children in adoptive American settings. *Developmental Psychology,* **18**, 595–99 (1982).

270. Ohwaki, S., & Stayton, S. The relation of length of institutionalization to the intellectual functioning of the profoundly retarded. *Child Development,* **49**, 105–109 (1978).

271. Yarrow, L. Separation from parents during early childhood. In M. Hoffman & L. Hoffman (Eds.), *Review of child development research.* Vol. 1. New York, Russell Sage, 1964.

272. Casler, L. The effects of extra tactual stimulation on a group of institutionalized infants. *Genetic Psychology Monographs* **71**, 137–75 (1965).

273. Sayegh, Y., & Dennis, W. The effect of supplementary experiences upon the development of infants in institutions. *Child Development,* **36**, 81–90 (1965).

274. Hunt, J. McV., Mohandessi, K., Ghodssi, M., & Akizama, M. The psychological

development of orphanage reared infants. *Genetic Psychology Monographs*, **94**, 177–226 (1976).

275. Paraskevopolous, J., & Hunt, J. McV. Object construction and imitation under differing conditions of rearing. *Journal of Genetic Psychology*, **119**, 301–321 (1971).

276. Tizard, B., & Rees, J. A comparison of the effect of adoption, restoration to the natural mother and continued institutionalization on the cognitive development of 4 year old children. In A. Clarke & A. Clarke (Eds.), *Early experience: Myth and evidence*. London, Open Book, 1976.

277. Wollins, M. The vulnerable child and the healing environment. In E. Anthony, C. Koupernik, & C. Chiland (Eds.), *The child in his family*. Vol. 4. New York, Wiley, 1978.

278. Mortimore, P. The study of institutions. *Human Relations*, **31**, 985–99 (1978).

279. Phillips, E., Wolf, M., Fixsen, D., & Bailey, J. The achievement place model: A community based family style behaviour modification program for predelinquents. In E. Ribes-Inesta & A. Bandura (Eds.), *Analysis of delinquency and aggression*. Hillsdale, NJ, Erlbaum, 1976.

280. Andrews, A., Blumenthal, J., Johnson, D., Kahn, A., Ferguson C., Lasater, T., Malone, P., & Wallace, D. The skills of mothering: A study of parent child development centers. *Monographs of the Society for Research in Child Development*, **47**, (198) (1982).

281. Cohen, H. B. Play – a community support system: Phase 1. In E. Ribes-Inesta & A. Bandura (Eds.), *Analysis of deliquency and aggression*. Hillsdale, NJ, Erlbaum, 1976.

282. Gonzalez, R. Mental health services for children in the Region of the Americas. *International Journal of Mental Health*, **7** (1–2), 39–48 (1978).

283. Olatawura, M. Mental health services for children in the African Region. *International Journal of Mental Health*, **7** (1–2), 34–38 (1978).

284. Walberg, H., Bole, R., & Waxman, A. School based family socialization and reading achievement in the inner city. *Psychology in the Schools*, **17**, 509–514 (1980).

285. Atkeson, B., & Forehand, R. Home based reinforcement programs designed to modify classroom behaviours: A review and methodological evaluation. *Psychological Bulletin*, **86**, 1298–1308 (1979).

286. Aarons, A., Hawes, H., & Gayton, J. *Child to child*. London, Macmillan, 1979.

287. Palmer, F., & Anderson, L. Early intervention treatments that have been tried, documented and assessed. In M. Begab, H. Haywood, & H. Barber (Eds.), *Psychosocial influences in retarded performance*. Vol. 2. Baltimore, MD, University Park Press, 1981.

288. Ramey, C., & Campbell, F. Early childhood education for psychosocially disadvantaged children. *American Journal of Mental Deficiency*, **83**, 645–48 (1979).

289. Williams, T. Infant development and supplemental care. A comparative review of basic and applied research. *Human Development*, **20**, 1–30 (1977).

290. Miller, L., & Dyer, J. Four preschool problems: Their dimensions and effects. *Monographs of the Society for Research in Child Development*, **40** (162) (1975).

291. Siegel, I., & Olmstead, P. Modification of cognitive skills among lower class Black children. In J. Hellmuth (Ed.), *The disadvantaged child*. Vol. 3. New York, Brunner/Mazel, 1970.

292. Lazar, I., & Darlington, R. Lasting effects of early education. *Monographs of the Society for Research in Child Development*, **47**, (195) (1982).

293. Bruner, J., & Connolly, K. Competence: The growth of the person. In K. Connolly & J. Bruner (Eds.), *The growth of competence*. New York, Academic Press, 1974.

294. Butkowsky, I., & Willows, D. Cognitive motivational characteristics of children ranging in reading ability. *Journal of Educational Psychology*, **72**, 408–422 (1980).

295. Parke, R. Children's home environments: Social and cognitive effects. In I. Altman & J. Wohlwill (Eds.), *Children and the environment*. New York, Plenum, 1978.

296. Abramson, L., Seligman, M., & Teasdale, J. Learned helplessness in humans: Critique and reformulation. *Journal of Abnormal Psychology*, **87**, 49–74 (1978).

297. Fowler, J., & Peterson, P. Increasing reading persistence and altering attributional style of learned helpless children. *Journal of Educational Psychology*, **73**, 251–60 (1981).

298. MacPhee, D., Ramey, C., & Yeates, K. The home environment and early mental development. In A. Gottfried (Ed.), *Home environment and early mental development*. New York, Academic Press, 1984.

299. Tan, E. Mental health services for children in the South East Asian and Western Pacific Regions. *International Journal of Mental Health*, **7** (1–2), 96–101 (1978).

300. Whitt, J., & Casey, P. The mother infant relationship and infant development: The effect of pediatric intervention. *Child Development*, **53**, 948–56 (1982).

301. Baasher, T. Mental health services for children in the Eastern Mediterranean Region. *International Journal of Mental Health*, **7**, (1–2), 49–64 (1978).

302. Minde, K. Child psychiatry in developing countries. *Journal of Child Psychology and Psychiatry*, **17**, 70–83 (1976).

303. Bronfenbrenner, U. *Is early intervention effective?* (DHEW Publication, No. 76–30025). Washington, DC, Department of Health, Education and Welfare, 1974.

304. Gray S., & Ruttle, K. The family oriented home visiting program: A longitudinal study. *Genetic Psychology Monographs*, **102**, 299–316 (1980).

4

Children in danger

Philip Graham

A conceptual framework
Traditionally in medicine, knowledge about harmful agents arises within the context of an accepted scheme for classifying disorders. For most diseases a single harmful agent, e.g. a virus, bacterium, or toxin, has been identified. This agent is usually necessary for the condition to occur, though actual appearance of the condition will depend on a host of other factors as well. Nonetheless, consideration of prevention and treatment focuses especially on the specific agent responsible. This model of causation has its limitations, but it has proved valuable and has produced clinical advances.

Classification of childhood behaviour and emotional problems is now more widely agreed upon than was previously the case. There are two rather similar major schemes for classification: the *International classification of diseases*, 9th edition (ICD-9) (1) and the *Diagnostic and statistical manual of mental disorders*, 3rd edition (DSM-III) (2). Both recognize the importance of considering separately a number of types of disorder in children – namely (in the case of ICD-9), mental disorders, intellectual and learning deficits, developmental delays, physical disabilities, and psychosocial disadvantages. Unfortunately, classification of child mental disorders does not usually lead to any clear-cut implications for causation, prevention, or treatment. The major types of problem behaviour in children (preschool management problems, emotional disorders, antisocial behaviour, psychoses, etc) do not have any single aetiology, and causation needs to be considered in a more complex manner, for a number of reasons (2, 3):

1. Known causative influences are not specific to particular disorders. For example, parental attitudes are likely to be of importance in a variety of conditions.

Dr Graham is with the Department of Child Psychiatry, Institute of Child Health, University of London, and the Hospital for Sick Children, Great Ormond St., London WC1, England.

2. Causative influences are usually multiple; thus, mental ill health in parents is often linked to parental marital disharmony.
3. There is often interaction among different causes, as there may well be between parental ill health and marital disharmony.
4. The effect of a cause is likely to be mitigated or exacerbated by the degree of vulnerability of the child. Such vulnerability may be genetically determined and expressed in the child's temperament; or it may be produced, for example, by a series of distressing events that have lowered the child's self-esteem.
5. The impact of a cause is also likely to depend on the manner in which it is perceived, both consciously and unconsciously, by the child. A child whose expectations include success in examinations is likely to be more disturbed by repeated failure than a child who did not expect to succeed. A boy whose parents have abandoned him will react differently if he sees his friends treated in the same way than if his experience appears to him to be unique.
6. There may well be a reverse interaction between a cause and its effects. For example, a child who reacts to emotional deprivation by violence to his parents or sibs may well find himself more emotionally deprived as a result of his reaction.

It may therefore be more appropriate to consider child psychological problems as determined in a rather complex, interactional manner than to use a simple, unidirectional, cause–effect model. Awareness of the possibility of complexity should not, however, produce defeatism with regard to change. If a stimulus is known to be noxious, then its removal is likely to be beneficial, and this holds in child behaviour as in medicine. The difference is that the results of interventions in child behaviour are likely to be less predictable and, it must be admitted, less immediately effective than is the case in medical conditions, because, in general, they are acting on complex systems. This certainly does not mean that interventions are valueless or, even less, that they should not be tried: there are many examples of successful interventions.

Situations dangerous for child mental health
Malnutrition
Throughout the world there are many millions of children whose diet is grossly deficient, who live in poverty-stricken circumstances, who are inadequately clothed, and housed in cramped quarters, and who receive little or no education. Children are living in such situations in developing countries with large rural populations, where the methods of agriculture are insufficient to sustain the size of population for which it must provide. Slums around large cities in economically under-developed countries are also settings for the co-existence of poverty and malnutrition. The *seiros* around Caracas, the *favellas* around Rio de Janeiro, and the

villas miserias around Buenos Aires are packed with children inadequately cared for or abandoned, who are living in unprotected circumstances and are highly vulnerable to the development of behavioural and emotional disorders.

Economic poverty is, in these circumstances, often linked to a breakdown of traditional patterns of family life. This is much more likely to occur in the slums of big cities than in rural areas: although the mortality rate of parents in starving populations in rural areas is high, patterns of extended family life usually ensure that orphaned or semi-orphaned children will be looked after by other family members.

There is controversy over the issue whether malnutrition can cause mental retardation and behavioural difficulties, some believing that the brain is specially protected against starvation and that, when cognitive deficits and abnormal behaviour are detectable in excess in malnourished populations, this is due to the accompanying social deprivation rather than to lack of food supply. The evidence that starvation alone can impair cognitive functioning to some degree is now reasonably convincing, however – but it is less certain whether behavioural abnormalities arise in this way. Richardson & co-workers (4) compared 6–10 year-old boys who had been admitted to hospital in the first two years of life in Jamaica because of kwashiorkor, marasmus, or marasmic kwashiorkor with their siblings and classroom controls. They found that boys who had experienced early malnutrition displayed numerous behavioural deficits in comparison with classroom controls, especially in classroom behaviour and in their peer relationships. These boys were less co-operative, had poorer memories, were easily distracted, and were less popular. There were, however, few differences in behaviour between these early malnourished children and their sibs. It is possible that the sibs suffered in early childhood from a lesser degree of malnutrition, insufficient to require hospital admission, but severe enough to result in later behavioural difficulties. Alternatively – and this is perhaps the more likely explanation – the behavioural difficulties may have been caused by the social factors operating within the family on both patients and their sibs, but not on classroom controls.

The malnourished child is particularly prone to infection, which itself may result in long-term neurological and mental impairment. Thus, children living in areas with borderline sufficient nutrition who are unprotected by vaccination and immunization are especially prone to conditions such as measles, encephalitis, tuberculosis, and poliomyelitis, all of which may result in chronic physical disability. And, as suggested later in this paper, children with physical handicaps are prone to develop behaviour and emotional problems, and this is particularly likely to occur when the organic lesion affects brain function. Rates of epilepsy, cerebral palsy, and other organic brain syndromes in malnourished populations in developing countries are not well recorded, but there is every reason to think that they are high (5).

Urban poverty

Those responsible for the upbringing of children (usually parents, but the task is often shared with others, especially other family members) need time, space, a sense of security, and the availability of help from others in the community if they are to carry out their task properly. If these positive attributes are lacking, then it becomes more likely that upbringing will be inadequate and that the children will develop emotional and behavioural disturbance. Clearly, many environmental factors are likely to affect whether the attributes necessary for good parenting are present or not. These factors do not operate directly on children: their impact is mediated through their effects on family life more generally. It has been well demonstrated (6) that, once family factors have been taken into account, the impact of other factors acting independently is very small or non-existent. What, then, are the other environmental factors acting upon families and indirectly upon children that endanger children? How do these factors operate, and what is the type of behavioural outcome that may be expected in their presence?

First, it is important to note that it has been demonstrated (7, 8) that children living in big cities in England and Norway are likely to show higher rates of behavioural disturbances than are children living in small towns or rural areas. There is no specific type of behavioural or emotional disturbance associated with living in a big city, though urban children do show an excess of both emotional and conduct disorders. Such comparative studies do not appear to have been carried out in developing countries; there is some suggestion (9), however, that the results would be similar.

Families living in big cities are apt to be disadvantaged in a number of ways. Often they enjoy less support from other family members: though families living in socially disorganized areas may be in touch with other family members, contact is often difficult, and support not forthcoming. Secondly, families living in cities have less access to outside space where their children can live and play in safety. Actually, density of population is not generally related to behavioural disturbance (10); but young children living in high-rise buildings with very restricted opportunities for play are more prone to disturbance, and their mothers more subject to depression (11). Thirdly, indoor space may be cramped and overcrowded so that parents lack privacy and become frustrated and irritable as a result. Overcrowding is associated with high rates of deviance, especially if accommodation and facilities have to be shared with non-family members (12). Fourthly, an urban family may be more likely to experience uncertainty regarding economic survival. This may also be the case in rural areas where agricultural production is close to a bare subsistence level and families are dependent upon favourable climatic conditions for survival; but it is perhaps a more common predicament among the poor living in big cities, whose ability to obtain jobs with any sort of secure tenure may be limited or non-existent. The relationship between parental unemployment and mental health in children is complex (*13*), but both direct and indirect effects of unemployment on rates of behavioural deviance have been demonstrated. Fifthly, families living in cities are dependent to a greater degree than those living in rural areas on the smooth working of complex institutions. A tap is a more secure source of water than a spring or well, but poor labour relations, inadequate technology, or undercapitalization may all result in a failure of a city's water supply, and in some parts of the world this is a frequent occurrence. Similarly, in rural areas there is little dependence on a public transportation system, whereas in cities the ability to buy food, get to work, get children to school, etc., may all depend on a satisfactorily functioning transport system. Deficiencies in any of these areas put parents under strain, and may make care of their children inadequate.

Three further points need to be made concerning children living in urban poverty. The first is that it is not just families living in the slum areas of cities whose children are disadvantaged; there are, in fact, few social-class differences in rates of childhood emotional and behavioural disorders. Slum children are most likely to display such problems, but *all* children in large cities must be regarded as living in potentially harmful circumstances. The second is that families continue to migrate to cities from rural areas despite the conditions they find when they arrive. There must therefore be a strong presumption that the economic and social circumstances in the rural areas from which they come are even more unsatisfactory. Thirdly, the slums of big cities must be seen as themselves products of an economic and social system that allows for uncontrolled movement of people in search of jobs and better living conditions. In considering preventive measures, one certainly needs to look at how the disadvantages of slum living can be ameliorated; but it is also necessary to examine how economic development can be achieved in ways less disruptive of family life than migration of rural people to the cities.

Environmental hazards

The most obvious adverse results of the development of modern technology on the health of children are in the areas of physical disability. In developed countries, accidents, of which from a third to a half are road traffic accidents, account for about half the mortality in children aged 1–14 years. Inappropriate diets, resulting in obesity and possibly in the development of allergic disorders, must also be viewed as exerting harmful effects on children's physical development.

Environmental hazards affecting child mental health are less well documented. Recently, however, there has been considerable concern about the effects of lead in the atmosphere on the intelligence and behavioural state of children. Children living near lead smelters or in houses with old, peeling, lead-based paint are at risk for the development of lead encephalopathy if their lead intake is high. It is somewhat less certain whether the mental development of children exposed to lower doses of lead are at risk (*14*), but some studies suggest that lead from gasoline may reduce intellectual functioning and, less probably, produce behaviour disorders. A number of countries have therefore embarked on national policies to reduce lead in gasoline and thus in the atmosphere.

Migration

Internal migration of families from rural to urban areas has already been mentioned, but movement of populations for other reasons is also a potential source of stress in children's lives. In some developed countries members of government departments, large business organizations, and armed services personnel are expected to be geographically mobile. Their families move with the job, and there is evidence that children who have to leave their schools and friends relatively frequently are unsettled by this experience.

On a much more widespread basis, patterns of employment that depend on migrant workers impose a different type of stress on children. Many Western European countries have encouraged the migration of male guest-workers from Southern European and North African countries, and these workers have often been separated from their families for months or years and had little contact with their children. Those given the right to settle temporarily or permanently with their families have encountered prejudice and discrimination. Nevertheless, rates of mental disturbance among children of migrants have in general not been found to be particularly high (*15, 16*); indeed, the self-protective mechanisms used by those living in communities in which they are exposed to hostile external influences may actually strengthen family ties.

Finally, one must mention migration of families produced by civil or international armed conflict. The impact of war on the lives of children may be profound as a result of the violent deaths of one or both parents, the type of uprooting that has occurred to many hundreds of thousands of children in Vietnam and the Middle East, or perhaps the less severe trauma experienced by children in areas where chronic civil conflict exists, as in Northern Ireland.

School factors

The influence of schools on rates of mental disturbance has been little studied until recently, as it has been assumed by most professionals that family factors and innate ability are of considerably greater importance. In recent years, however, there has been increasing interest in the possibility that schools vary in their capacity both to promote and to inhibit healthy psychosocial development, and studies have now demonstrated that such variation does indeed exist.

There are considerable methodological problems in the study of school influences. Parents who send their children to schools with a deservedly bad reputation for high rates of delinquency may, in addition, be providing inadequate care at home; and if the outcome is poor, it may be difficult to determine how much is attributable to the school and how much to home influences. In order to overcome this problem, it is necessary to control the home factors when examining differences in outcome among schools. The measurement of what goes on inside a school is also problematic. It is sometimes difficult to obtain permission to study the internal organization and policy of schools. If access is gained, the quantification of potentially important factors such as the quality of communication, the level of pastoral care, etc., poses further problems.

Nevertheless, methods now exist to measure such aspects of school functioning. It seems that, at least in London schools (*17*), academic attainment, behavioural and emotional disorders, and truancy are related to certain specific factors, such as the emphasis given to an academic approach, the control by reward rather than by punishment, and the degree to which responsibility is shared among the pupils. By contrast, factors such as size of the school, pupil/teacher ratio, and the emphasis placed on pastoral care are not related to outcome.

Family breakdown

Before considering factors within families that put children in danger, it is appropriate to discuss the care provided for children for whom family care has broken down or for whom it has never been available. For children abandoned at birth or for whom it becomes clear in the first few weeks of life that parental care is inadequate, a whole childhood may be spent in institutions. Others whose parents die, become ill, or unable to look after their children for other reasons may similarly spend a substantial period of time in an orphanage.

It has now been well demonstrated that institutional care, even in small children's homes, let alone the large impersonal institutions in existence in many developing and some developed countries, is an inadequate substitute for family care for the great majority of children (*18*). A small minority of antisocial children for whom parental care has broken down in mid- or late childhood may not be able to cope with the emotional demands of family life. For all other children, but especially for those whose care breaks down in infancy, substitute family care is superior to institutional care.

Adoption or, as second best, long-term fostering in carefully selected families therefore provides the most suitable type of family care if the extended family is unable to assume this responsibility. The evidence suggests that early-adopted children have no more than the expected rate of behaviour and emotional problems.

Where adoption is not culturally acceptable, resort to institutional care is inevitable. It is therefore important to note that the organization of institutions and various other factors related to them are important predictors of outcome. It has been demonstrated that avoidance of hierarchy plus personalized care for children – caretakers being assigned to particular children – produces better-adjusted, brighter children. In general, such factors are more likely to be present when the size of the institution is relatively small and when the ratio of caretakers to children is reasonably high. This means that good substitute care for children is inevitably expensive.

Family care

In infancy and the early years of childhood, children's emotional needs, throughout the world, are met within families or by extended family care. Later in childhood, extrafamilial influences encountered in school and in the neighbourhood gain in importance, but the influence of the family of origin on individual development remains vital throughout adolescence and, in many cultures, well into adult life. When children's needs for emotional development are not met within the family, they are therefore in danger of faulty personality development. What, then, are these needs?

The first, and perhaps the most important, is a continuous caring relationship by the same adults – usually, though not necessarily, the children's parents – over the entire period of childhood. Breaks in care or transfers of care that result in loss of parental figures act to the disadvantage of children. It has been well demonstrated that child care can be effectively shared among a limited number of family members, and that relatively brief separations from family figures, such as may occur when a mother goes out to work or a child goes to stay with a familiar relative, may actually promote child development in a healthy manner. But prolonged separations, especially if they involve institutionalization with unfamiliar figures, are certainly upsetting in the short term, and may have long-term consequences on children's personality growth. Even short separations for hospital care may have persisting deleterious effects (19).

Secondly, it is important that attitudes and behaviour toward children involve warmth, affection, and emphasis on the child's positive attributes. Children brought up by parents who are overly critical or punitive are more likely to develop both emotional difficulties and behaviour problems (20).

Thirdly, children need to have defined for them reasonably clear-cut boundaries for their behaviour. If children are not brought up to know what is and is not permitted, they will later have difficulty in coping with the limitations the wider society places upon them. This means that parents have to accept their role as boundary-keepers, using, to the extent possible, positive means to help children remain within acceptable limits rather than punishment for transgression. It also means that parents have to acknowledge their supervisory role; and this may be difficult, for they may be confused regarding the setting of limits within the context of a loving relationship.

Fourthly, there is a need for children to have time and space for exploration. This requirement is easily met in most rural areas in developing countries, but is much less easily satisfied in urban areas in developed countries. Physical exploration, moreover, is not enough: there is also a need for children to explore and develop the use of language in relation to their environment. This they are likely to be able to do only if there are adults around who can provide a rich and stimulating language environment, so that the child's own inherent language ability can be stimulated to develop to its fullest extent.

These needs will be met only if responsible family members are flexible enough to be sensitive to the growing child's changing requirements. Obviously, the control the teenager needs is of a different quality from that required by a preschool child, but some parents find it difficult to adapt to children's changing needs.

Finally, parents need also to act as mediators between the child and the external world. Friends, school, and the local neighbourhood provide opportunities for growth that are not available within the family; but some children are too shy or withdrawn to benefit, and others impinge violently on the wider environment so that they meet with rejection. In both instances parents need to act as mediators to ensure that the relationship between the child and others around him in the world beyond the family is satisfactory.

As already stated, children are likely to be in danger if family care is not able to meet these various needs. There are many situations in which this is likely to occur, and they can be conveniently summarized under five main headings.

1. *Parental death.* The death of at least one parent is a relatively common event in rural areas in developing countries, where, for example, every childbirth puts the life of a woman at significant risk and where serious infectious disease is still common. Children who have lost one parent through death are at somewhat increased risk for the development of emotional or behavioural disorder, but this is less likely to occur if their care is taken over by substitute family members. The reactions of children to parental death are determined primarily by the reactions of those around them (*21*).

2. *Parental physical illness.* Serious life-threatening illness in parents occurs much more commonly in developing than in developed countries. Children's lives may be affected in a variety of ways. Girls, for example, may have to take over many domestic duties, and indeed look after their mothers if they, the mothers, become incapacitated. When one or both parents suffer chronic illness, this may drastically affect the economic level at which the family can function, which may also have a major impact on a child's life.

3. *Disharmony of family relationships,* with associated quarrelling and family tension, is probably the most common source of stress for children in the developed world. There is ample evidence (*22*) that children brought up in such circumstances are particularly prone to conduct disturbances, but they may display

other problems. Marital disharmony is apt to be associated with inconsistency of discipline. Parents who are not meeting each other's emotional needs are likely to be uncommonly irritable with their children; sometimes they turn to their children in an inappropriate manner for comfort and caring.

In view of the impact of family disharmony on the frequency of childhood behaviour and emotional problems, it is not surprising that parental separation and divorce are linked to high rates of mental health problems in children. Children of all ages are likely to be adversely affected, boys being somewhat more at risk than girls. There is no clear-cut evidence that, from the point of view of the children, it is better for discordant, quarrelling parents to stay together or to part, although there is some suggestion that separation may be associated with a slightly better outcome for the mother. What does seem clear is that if parents who separate can make amicable arrangements regarding subsequent child care, and if they are able to communicate without bitterness and to avoid denigrating each other after separation has occurred, the outcome for the children is more satisfactory (23).

4. *Mental illness in one or both parents* is also linked to high rates of emotional problems in children (24). The most common form of mental health problem in parents to affect children is the depressive reaction, often accompanied by anxiety and irritability. Weissman (25) has shown how such reactions impair the capacity of mothers to cope with child-rearing tasks. In terms of understanding the factors putting children of depressed mothers at risk, it is, of course, important to take into account the stresses that may have been responsible for the mother's depression in the first place.

Psychotic disorders in parents are, perhaps paradoxically, less likely to affect children's mental health development adversely. This is probably partly because the parent's disorder is generally perceived in illness terms and leads less frequently to parental disharmony, and partly because the well parent may be able to cope satisfactorily with the children and to meet their needs. If the morbid behaviour displayed by psychotic parents involves the children, e.g. if a father believes his children are trying to poison him, then adverse effects on child development are more apt to occur.

There is a strong link between personality disorder in parents, especially if this is of an aggressive, antisocial type, and the development of behaviour problems in children. This effect is probably partly genetically determined and partly fostered by inappropriate upbringing. Violent parents are more likely to be inconsistent in their upbringing, to frustrate their children's needs, and to provide inappropriate models for imitation and identification. Aggressive parents are, of course, also more likely to have marriages that are disharmonious and otherwise unsatisfactory; it is often difficult to disentangle the adverse effects on children of family relationships and parental personality problems.

5. Finally, one must note that some children living in families in which both parents are still alive, neither parent is physically or mentally ill, and the parental marital relationship is satisfactory are nevertheless at risk by virtue of *inappropriate upbringing*. In some circumstances it would seem that this situation has arisen because of severe social stress acting upon parents in ways described above. A mother or father may react to unemployment, financial hardship, poor housing, etc., not by developing mental illness, but by impaired parenting capacity.

Ignorance and lack of experience are further reasons for unsatisfactory parenting. Many parents, especially those brought up in isolated families with few children around, may have very little experience in child rearing, and preparation for parenthood is often low on the list of priorities in school curricula. Parents who have experienced unsatisfactory parenting in their own childhood may also find it difficult to rear their children with warmth and empathy even if they are in no way suffering from personality disorders.

Personal factors within children

So far, in considering children in danger, we have examined factors in the wider environment and in the family. It is important to acknowledge, however, that children may be rendered vulnerable to stress by factors within themselves. Children may be in danger not just because of the influences acting upon them, but also because of the attributes they themselves possess.

Genetic vulnerability

There is some evidence from both adoption studies (26) and twin studies (27) that some children may be more at risk for the development of mental health problems if they are genetically vulnerable. It is certainly the impression of parents that children differ in their inherited capacity to respond to stress, and scientific evidence supports this view.

The most significant phenotypic manifestation of inherited vulnerability is probably the child's temperament. Evidence exists (28, 29) to suggest that temperamental characteristics may determine whether, faced with environmental adversity, a child develops behaviour problems and, moreover, if a problem does develop, the type of reaction the child will display. There is also some evidence (30) that genetic factors determine such characteristics.

Physical disorders in children

It is well established (31) that children with chronic physical handicaps are about twice as likely to display behaviour and emotional disorders than are children in the general population. This effect is probably mediated by alterations in parental child-rearing, self-concept, and the prejudice and discrimination physically handicapped children receive in the community, especially at school. Certain handicaps such as obesity and facial deformity are more apt to elicit teasing and bullying than other disabilities.

Children suffering from physical disorders affecting brain functioning are particularly prone to develop mental health problems (32). For example, children with uncomplicated epilepsy are four or five times more apt to display such problems as children in the general population. It is probable that, in these cases, disturbances in brain functioning result in a failure to integrate new experiences and that this, in itself, results in the child's experiencing additional frustration in social and learning situations.

Coping capacity

When faced with stressful situations, children vary in their capacity to develop strategies to achieve mastery. The factors leading to successful coping are poorly understood. It seems likely that overprotected children who have been given inadequate opportunities to achieve independence are at special risk. Some parents and teachers are more consciously aware of their responsibility to teach children to cope with the life problems facing them, and this may also be of importance in how well or poorly children subsequently overcome the inevitable hazards they meet at school, in employment, and in their personal relationships in the wider world.

Children in danger: a global perspective

Much of the research work summarized above has been conducted in developed countries, but an attempt has been made to provide information that would be most relevant to children living in economically underdeveloped regions of the world. How far is it possible to generalize from developed to developing countries in child mental health?

The World Health Organization (WHO) has stimulated individuals, or groups of individuals, in eight different countries to collect information concerning prevalence rates, service provision, and training of personnel in child mental health. The data obtained from this exercise, which was carried out in Costa Rica, Egypt, France, Greece, Indonesia, Nigeria, Sri Lanka and Thailand, has been summarized by Sartorius & Graham (33).

Despite wide variations in size of population, level of economic development, predominant religious belief, level of literacy, etc., it was clear that the children in these countries responded in remarkably similar ways to the stresses they faced. There was generally a disappointing lack of epidemiological data documenting rates of behavioural and emotional disorders, epilepsy, and mental retardation. Many of the major stresses such as family disruption and pressure for academic achievement were present everywhere. Anecdotally, certain childhood problems such as suicide and attempted suicide were found to be increasing. There was little or no evidence of culture-specific syndromes.

Health service resources were everywhere regarded as in too short supply to provide adequate prevention and treatment in child mental health, and training in this area was also universally regarded as inadequate. This impression is confirmed by the findings of a WHO-supported study (34) in which it was demonstrated that primary health workers had difficulty in identifying child mental health problems even in children attending their clinics.

Primary health care: existing patterns

In rural areas in developing countries, the person concerned with assessing and treating health problems is generally a village health worker with very limited training, though often with a great deal of experience. His or her training will be in measures necessary to improve hygiene and diet, to prevent specific diseases, and to assess and treat common disorders. A primary care physician will be available for referral of cases, either on the spot or at a referral centre.

In big cities in developing countries, the pattern will vary. The main tasks of prevention will probably be in the hands of community nurses. Assessment and treatment of common disorders may be carried out by such a nurse or by a primary care physician. In either event, the time available for each personal intervention is generally very limited. In cities, such care may be given in a community health centre or in the office of a physician. A substantial component of primary health care in cities is also delivered in accident and emergency or outpatient departments of general hospitals.

In most developed countries, preventive activities in childhood are likely to be shared between community nurses and physicians, community nurses playing an especially important part in the first five years of life. Differences between urban and rural areas in the delivery of health care are less marked, although they certainly exist. The delivery of health care takes place in health centres or the offices of physicians. In big cities, however, hospital outpatient services also provide a substantial proportion of primary health care, especially to the poorer segments of the population.

The professional training of the physician involved in the delivery of primary health care to children in developed countries varies. In some countries, as in the USSR or USA, the physician will be trained as a paediatrician; in others, such as the United Kingdom, he or she will be a family practitioner dealing with health problems of people of all ages; in yet others, there is variation within the country. Whatever their training and background, such physicians are probably able to devote more time to each problem than is the case in developing countries; nevertheless, the allocation of time, perhaps 10 to 15 minutes maximum for each child, is usually not generous (35).

120   *Philip Graham*

It is important to re-emphasize that the tasks necessary for the achievement of good health are by no means all the responsibility of professional health workers. Quite apart from parents and other family members whose care is basic and essential to good health, other professionals may be heavily involved. For instance, teachers as well as nurses may instruct children in principles of hygiene and diet, and may be involved in identifying common health problems and suggesting remedies. Especially in rural areas in developing countries, traditional healers play a large part in the primary treatment of disorders. In the cities of both developed and developing countries, social workers involved in the protection of children for whom parental care has broken down or is totally inadequate will be involved in assessment and decision making of great relevance to health, especially to healthy mental development.

Requirements for better delivery of mental health care
In both developing and developed countries it is apparent that much greater emphasis is given to physical than to mental health problems in both the training and the practice of those involved in primary health care. The most cursory examination of primary health care manuals and textbooks makes this apparent. It is also the case that mental health problems are widely prevalent, are frequently brought to the attention of primary care practitioners, are often not identified, and are often inadequately assessed and treated.

There would appear to be three main avenues open to improvement in this unsatisfactory situation, each of which has research implications:

- The primary health care worker needs re-orientation to include mental health care in his or her purview.
- There is a need for improvement in knowledge to ensure that necessary tasks can be carried out economically and effectively.
- Techniques for widespread dissemination of existing knowledge, with continuing evaluation of delivery of care, need to be developed.

Redefinition of tasks and boundaries
Understandably in developing, and perhaps less understandably in developed countries, training in health care has, until now, heavily emphasized the physical or somatic aspects of disease in children. Little instruction is usually given on the importance of psychological or social factors in the development of physical disorders, or on the more purely mental problems often encountered in practice. It is striking how little attention is given to mental health in the content of examinations and in the evaluation of courses. Consequently, health practitioners do not perceive themselves to be the right people to deal with these problems and, when faced with them, usually feel inadequate, and may respond with a lack of

sympathy or inappropriate advice. It is common for a physician to say to a mother with a seriously disabled child, 'There is nothing wrong with your child,' when what he means is that he can detect no physical abnormality or sign of physical disease and suspects that the symptoms have a psychological cause.

It would be of some value to establish among primary health care workers and physicians the extent to which they perceive their role to include the assessment and treatment of mental health problems. The development of simple attitude questionnaires, including questions on the degree to which practitioners think certain problems (both physical and mental) fall within their province, would not be a difficult matter; and questions could also be asked on the frequency with which practitioners think such problems are brought to them and how competent they feel themselves to be in dealing with them. Such research could be carried out relatively easily as special projects by medical, psychology, or social-work students.

Increased knowledge
Epidemiological studies
One of the reasons why health care practitioners are reluctant to develop skills in the assessment and management of mental health problems is a widespread belief that, especially in rural areas, such difficulties do not exist, or exist only rarely. This is also one of the reasons, although perhaps not the most important, why it would be helpful to conduct epidemiological studies of mental health problems to establish, to a much greater degree than has been the case hitherto, the incidence, prevalence, and short-term course of disorders. Certainly, countries envisaging putting substantial extra resources into child mental health would be well advised to embark on epidemiological studies at the same time as they increase such resources. Information about general population incidence and prevalence of mental health problems and the frequency of links between physical disorders and developmental, learning, and emotional disorders is of special relevance to primary health workers, who see such a high proportion of the child population.

Such studies need not be expensive, especially if students engaged in projects are used as interviewers (though there is certainly a need for such students to be well supervised). In both developing and developed countries, it is sometimes the case that students in psychology and social administration departments are involved in carrying out projects of little relevance to the needs of the population. The opportunities for questionnaire design, acquisition of interviewing skills, gaining of community experience, and data analysis that epidemiological studies provide make them excellent learning tools. Ideally, such studies should test hypotheses, involving, for example, comparisons of rates among groups, or the investigation of background social and psychological factors related to a particular physical problem.

Development of brief assessment and treatment procedures
As already indicated, primary health care workers are handicapped by a lack of agreed-upon assessment and short-term treatment procedures. A start has been made on the development of such procedures with the production by the WHO South-East Asia Regional Office (SEARO) child mental health manuals (36). These consist of simple statements concerning the emotional needs of children of different ages. They then go on to describe in simple language the mental health problems children present and to provide practical advice on how to deal with them. Separate manuals have been developed for primary health care workers, teachers, child-care workers, and primary care physicians. Although it has been reported that these manuals are valuable in practice, they should be evaluated in a systematic manner and modified as needed.

Development of brief treatment procedures
The SEARO manuals are of particular relevance to those working in developing countries. In developed countries there is an equally great need to produce guidelines, suitable for general practitioners able to make a somewhat greater investment of time, on the management of mental health problems. At the moment, although primary care practitioners in developed countries are increasingly beginning to recognize their responsibility for mental health problems, they lack acceptable, short-term treatment measures for dealing with problems such as, for example, minor depressive reactions, sleep disorders, appetite problems, and hyperactivity. In some cases it would be inappropriate for practitioners to take a symptomatic approach to treatment when presented with problems such as these; but there are many reasonably rapid and useful symptomatic measures, developed by child psychiatrists and psychologists, that could be adapted for use in the primary health care setting and tested and evaluated there. Similarly, non-symptomatic measures, such as counselling, are often poorly applied in primary care, probably at least partly because those who are most expert in such measures have given little thought to their adaptation for use within the limited time available in primary care work.

Effects of schooling
The importance for the mental health of children of aspects of the expanding educational system has already been stressed. It would be unfortunate if any impression were given that educational expansion is not of clear benefit to developing countries involved in this effort, but the fact remains that it is becoming increasingly evident that there are many casualties as a result of the new systems. There is a need to investigate the experience of low educational performance despite adequate learning opportunity, to determine to what extent it is inevitable for this situation to be accompanied by feelings of low self-esteem and

worthlessness. Apparently high rates of suicide and attempted suicide among unsuccessful students, anecdotally reported from some countries, require investigation, because the appearance of such extreme self-destructiveness suggests the presence of a much more prevalent, similar phenomenon of lesser severity.

Research on care delivery

There is already evidence suggesting that the addition of a psychosocial dimension to treatment measures applied to malnourished children admitted to hospital shortens the length of time needed for treatment and reduces the risk of relapse (*37, 38*). There is a need to carry out, or build upon, work examining whether home visiting and other community measures applied to families at risk can reduce the subsequent rates of malnutrition among children. Also needed is an examination of ways in which communities containing a significant number of mothers whose level of care appears inadequate can be encouraged to develop self-help methods to improve the outcome of children at risk, and of ways in which counselling on home care, intellectual stimulation, and diet can be included in the advice given by primary care workers in areas where malnutrition is common.

As already indicated, the poor mental health of children and families living in appalling circumstances in the slums and poorer quarters of large cities cannot usefully be seen in isolation from the social and economic conditions producing such circumstances. Nevertheless, it is important that the health and social-welfare resources that are available for prevention and alleviation of different types of disorder be used to best advantage. There are already many experimental attempts to do just this, and good practices in existing forms of delivery of mental health care to seriously socially deprived children should be documented and disseminated.

Certain measures would seem to offer economical and effective means of delivering mental health care. First, close cooperation and joint training of health and social-welfare workers might ensure that when a professional worker of either discipline was in contact with a family, he or she could give appropriate advice concerning a broad range of measures, e.g. the social-welfare worker could give advice on immunization and accident prevention, and the health worker, on the importance for children of continuity of care. Second, greater emphasis on the development of self-help skills and mutual community support as part of the function of health workers would probably result in improved mental health care. Again, from a research point of view, the need would seem to be to take existing models of practice, ensure adequate description and definition, and then undertake evaluation, for example, by comparison with an area in which a different approach has been used.

In many countries where family care has broken down, there is no substitute for institutional care, e.g., in countries in which foster care and adoption are not acceptable practices. The lack of acceptability of substitute family care needs closer examination in these countries. For the child, such attitudes (though doubtless strongly rooted in concerns regarding biological and economic inheritance) probably have disastrous consequences. There is a need to study, perhaps in association with religious leaders, ways in which such cultural beliefs might be interpreted in a manner more helpful to the upbringing and personality development of children.

In countries where institutionalization of abandoned children is common, there is a need to determine the appropriateness of institutional practices and, when possible, to establish a set of guidelines for the use of the professionals involved in providing services. These might cover levels of staffing, attachment of individual workers to particular children, maintenance of contact with original families, transition to adult life, record-keeping, etc.

In developed countries the fact that the brightest students take academic courses and examinations whose content bears no relationship whatever to tasks of family life and parenthood means that such adult activities tend to be devalued or regarded as not amenable to instruction. Of course, most preparation for parenthood does take place in the home, but this does not mean that the school should not impart knowledge concerning health care and the needs of children. Opportunities to do so are rarely fully seized, and there is often rather inadequate input from health care workers into the curriculum to ensure that what is taught is accurate and relevant. The content of educational curricula for elementary school-children should be examined and evaluated with this in mind.

References

1. World Health Organization. *Mental disorders: Glossary and guide to their classification in accordance with the Ninth Revision of the International Classification of Diseases.* Geneva, World Health Organization, 1978.

2. American Psychiatric Association. *Diagnostic and statistical manual of mental disorders* (3rd ed.). Washington, DC, American Psychiatric Association, 1980.

3. Rutter, M., Shaffer, D., & Shepherd, M. *A multi-axial classification of child psychiatric disorders.* Geneva, World Health Organization, 1975.

4. Richardson, S. A., Birch, H. G., Grabie, E., & Yoder, K. The behaviour of children in school who were severely malnourished in the first two years of life. *Journal of Health and Social Behaviour,* **13**, 276–84 (1972).

5. Graham, P. J. Epidemiological approaches to child mental health in developing countries. In E. F. Purcell (Ed.), *Psychopathology of children and youth: A cross-cultural perspective.* New York, Josiah Macy, Jr., Foundation, 1980.

6. Rutter, M., & Quinton, D. Psychological disorder – Ecological factors and concepts of causation. In H. McGurk (Ed.), *Ecological factors in human development.* Amsterdam, North Holland, 1977.

7. Rutter, M., Cox, A., Tupling, L., Berger, M., & Yule, W. Attainment and adjustment in two geographical areas. I. The prevalence of psychiatric disorder. *British Journal of Psychiatry*, **126**, 493–509 (1975).

8. Lavik, N. J. Urban–rural differences in rates of disorder: A comparative psychiatric population study of Norwegian adolescents. In P. J. Graham (Ed.), *Epidemiological approaches in child psychiatry*. London, Academic Press, 1977. Pp. 233–51.

9. Minde, K. Child psychiatry in developing countries. *Journal of Child Psychology and Psychiatry*, **77**, 79–84 (1976).

10. Quinton, D. Cultural and community influences. In M. Rutter (Ed.), *Scientific foundations of developmental psychiatry*. London, Heinemann. Pp. 77–91.

11. Richman, N. Behaviour problems in pre-school children: Family and social factors. *British Journal of Psychiatry*, **131**, 523–27 (1977).

12. Mitchell, R. E. Some social implications of high density housing. *American Sociological Review*, **36**, 18–29 (1971).

13. Madge, N. Unemployment and its effects on children. *Journal of Child Psychology and Psychiatry*, **24**, 311–19 (1983).

14. Smith, M., Delves, T., Lansdown, R., Clayton, B., & Graham, P. The effects of lead on urban children. The Institute of Child Health/Southampton Study. *Developmental Medicine and Child Neurology*, **25**, Suppl. 47 (1983).

15. Rutter, M., Yule, W., Berger, M., Yule, B., Morton, J., & Bagley, C. Children of West Indian immigrants. I. Rates of behavioural deviance and of psychiatric disorder. *Journal of Child Psychology and Psychiatry*, **15**, 241–62 (1974).

16. Steinhausen, H.-C., & Remschmidt, H. Child and family psychopathology of migrants. In M. H. Schmidt & H. Remschmidt (Eds.), *Epidemiological approaches in child psychiatry, II*. Stuttgart, Georg Thieme Verlag, 1983. Pp. 185–95.

17. Rutter, M., Maughan, B., Mortimore, P., & Ouston, J. *Fifteen thousand hours*. London, Open Books, 1979.

18. Wolkind, S. W. Sex differences in the aetiology of antisocial disorders in children in long-term residential care. *British Journal of Psychiatry*, **125**, 125–30 (1974).

19. Douglas, J. Early hospital admission and later disturbances of behaviour and learning. *Developmental Medicine and Child Neurology*, **17**, 456–80 (1975).

20. Rutter, M. Other family influences. In M. Rutter & L. Hersov (Eds.), *Child psychiatry: Modern approaches*. Oxford, Blackwell Scientific Publications, 1977.

21. Black, D. The bereaved child – Annotation. *Journal of Child Psychology and Psychiatry*, **19**, 289–92 (1978).

22. Rutter, M., & Giller, H. *Juvenile delinquency: Trends and perspectives*. Harmondsworth, Penguin Books, 1983.

23. Wallerstein, J., & Kelly, J. Children and disorders. In J. Noshpitz (Ed.), *Basic handbook of child psychiatry*. Vol. 4. New York, Basic Books, 1979.

24. Rutter, M. *Children of sick parents*. London, Oxford University Press, 1966.

25. Weissman, M. M., & Paykel, E. *The depressed woman: A study of social relationships.* Chicago, University of Chicago Press, 1974.

26. Hutchings, B., & Mednick, S. Registered criminality in the adoptive and biological parents of registered male adoptees. In S. Mednick, F. Schulsinger, J. Higgins, &

B. Bell (Eds.), *Genetics, environment and psychopathology.* Amsterdam, North Holland. Pp. 215–27.

27.   Graham, P. J., & Stevenson, J. A twin study of genetic influences on behavioural deviance. *Journal of the American Academy of Child Psychiatry,* **24**, 33–41 (1985).

28.   Thomas, A., Chess, S., & Birch, H. G. *Temperament and behavior disorders in children.* New York, New York University Press, 1968.

29.   Graham, P., Rutter, M., & George, S. Temperamental characteristics as predictors of behaviour disorders in children. *American Journal of Orthopsychiatry,* **43**, 328–39 (1973).

30.   Rutter, M., Karn, S., & Birch, H. G. Genetic and environmental factors in the development of primary reaction patterns., *British Journal of Social and Clinical Psychology,* **2**, 161–73 (1967).

31.   Rutter, M., Graham, P., & Yule, W. *A neuropsychiatric study in childhood. Clinics in developmental medicine,* Nos. 35/36. London, Heinemann Medical Books, 1970.

32.   Graham, P., & Rutter, M. Organic brain dysfunction and child psychiatric disorder. *British Medical Journal,* **3**, 695–700 (1968).

33.   Sartorius, N., & Graham, P. Child mental health: Experience in eight countries. *WHO Chronicle,* **38** (5), 208–211 (1984).

34.   Giel, R., De Arango, M., & Climent, C. Childhood mental disorders in primary health care in poor developing countries. *Pediatrics,* **68**, 677–83 (1981).

35.   Graham, P. Primary health care in child psychiatry. *Acta Psychiatrica Scandinavica,* **62**, Suppl. 285, pp. 48–53 (1980).

36.   World Health Organization. *A manual on child mental health and psychosocial development.* Parts I–IV (SEA/Ment/65–68). New Delhi, WHO Regional Office for South-East Asia, 1982.

37.   Cravioto, J., & Arrieta, R. Stimulation and mental development of malnourished infants. *Lancet,* **2**, 899 (1979).

38.   Ramsay, F. C. Nutrition indicators and the Barbados school child: Nutrition intervention program. In US Department of Health, Education and Welfare, *Evaluation of child health services* (DHEW Pub. No. 78–1066). Washington, DC, US Government Printing Office, 1978. Pp. 169–92.

5

Adolescent health care and disease prevention in the Americas

Beatrix A. Hamburg

In dealing with the subject of adolescence, problems of definition immediately arise. Some social scientists view adolescence as a recent cultural invention of the Industrial Revolution devised primarily as a lengthy transitional stage to keep young persons out of the labour market (1). This is not an adequate explanation. In a myriad of guises, adolescence is a significant developmental transition, which is recognized in all types of cultures, and whose evolutionary roots have been clearly described in systematic studies of non-human primates.[1]

Adolescence has two major aspects, a biological one, and a sociocultural one. The biological changes of puberty mark the initiation or lower end of the adolescent period; the upper end or termination of the adolescence is marked by the induction of the individual into adult social roles and responsibilities. As a society becomes more and more complex, the timing of assumption of adult roles is increasingly delayed. In the most complex, affluent, and industrialized nations, the age limits defining adolescence may extend from age 10 through 20 or more years of age. The extension of time is largely at the upper end of adolescence and is due to postponement of assumption of adult roles; but in these same countries, there is an extension at the lower end as well.

The rate of biological maturation and the changes of puberty are related to the nutritional and overall health status of the individual, and studies in several Western nations have demonstrated a secular trend toward lowering the age of menarche (the sentinel event of pubertal maturation) by three months per decade (2). Under optimal health conditions, the average age of menarche is at about twelve and a half years; in developing nations and/or under conditions of poor health and nutritional deprivation, however, the typical age of menarche may be as late as 16 years. Whether puberty occurs early or late, the sequence and the nature of the biological changes are virtually identical across cultures.

Dr Hamburg is Professor of Psychiatry and Pediatrics, Mount Sinai School of Medicine, 1 Gustave L. Levy Place, New York, NY 10029, USA.

Clearly, chronological age definitions of adolescence are of only minimal usefulness; biological definitions that refer to maturational level are more informative. The biological changes of puberty endow the individual with the physical capability to perform adult functions. Among females, this refers chiefly to the constellation of anatomical and physiological changes that make child-bearing and lactation possible. Among males, in addition to the development of secondary sex characteristics, pubertal changes involve anatomical and physiological changes in respiratory, circulatory, and muscular systems that lead to remarkable increases in strength and endurance. There are also hormonal changes that enhance sexuality and aggressiveness.

When postpubertal youths with adult capacities are retained in childlike roles for lengthy periods of time, the developmental phase of adolescence assumes great prominence, and social inventions are required to cope with the challenges this presents. Indeed, many of the problems regarding adolescents in developed nations result from premature adoption of adult behaviours that are forbidden to adolescents, such as smoking, drinking, and sexual activity. The special opportunities of a lengthy adolescent period for fostering healthy development need more attention.

In the developing nations and under conditions of deprivation, adolescence may be very brief. In fact, the brevity of the transition to adulthood may lead the casual observer to believe that adolescence does not exist at all. None the less, however brief the duration of adolescence, most cultures do take ritual note of its achievement and endorse the entry into adulthood, often by explicit rites of puberty. These may include marriage of the girls and inclusion of the boys in adult work, war, or the political life of the village and/or moving them out of the mother's house to all-male quarters.

In North America, on the basis of data drawn mostly from the United States, the age range for adolescence is often put at ages 10–20 years; most of the data from Latin American nations report on ages 15–19 years.

Such categorizations in data-reporting are, in fact, social indicators: they tell us for which conditions and for which segments of the population there is public concern. For example, it is worth noting that it is only within the past decade that the US National Center for Health Statistics has collected and reported separate data for the 10–15 year age-group, and then only for selected conditions – accidents, drug use, smoking, alcohol use, and pregnancy. There was, however, a considerable lag between the time at which these problems became notably prominent in young adolescents under 15 years of age and the decision to begin to report separately for that age-group.

This is a serious matter, for, until appropriate diagnostic categories and age brackets are established for systematic data collection, it is impossible to trace the trends in the spread of important problems or to evaluate the efficacy of

Table 1. *Youth population in Americas, 1980 (selected countries)*

Country	Total population (millions)	% 15–19 years	% under 15
Argentina	28.7	8.2	27.6
Bolivia	6.4	10.3	43.8
Brazil	137.2	10.6	37.5
Chile	12.1	9.8	31.2
Colombia	28.7	11.3	37.2
Cuba	10.2	11.5	26.4
Ecuador	9.4	10.6	44.2
El Salvador	5.6	10.7	44.6
Mexico	80.5	11.2	42.9
Paraguay	3.7	10.8	41.7
Peru	20.3	10.9	41.4
Uruguay	3.0	8.2	27.0
USA	234.5	7.5	22.9
Venezuela	18.4	10.6	41.0

Source: Demographic indicators of countries: estimates and projections as assessed in 1980 (ST/ESA/SER. A/82), New York, United Nations Department of International Economic and Social Affairs, 1982.

intervention efforts. In countries where the menarche comes late and adolescence is short, the 15–19 year-old age bracket for national data collection may be suitable; but surveillance in other ways should be maintained to assure that important trends or conditions are not overlooked, and that the establishment of appropriate new reporting categories is not unduly delayed.

These issues become relevant in relation to the rapid social changes that characterize many of the developing nations. It is probable that some of these social changes are having, or will have, significant (sometimes drastic) effects on the physical and mental health of adolescents. There are important social changes that relate to urbanization, industrialization, large-scale migration, prolongation of education, unemployment, a vast increase in scale of the community of reference, and greater cultural heterogeneity. Taken together, these factors tend to weaken and even rupture the fabric of traditional cultures and to attenuate their socializing, orienting, and supportive functions. The weakening or loss of traditional family roles may have a critical impact on adolescents, especially when there are no substitutes for the vital family functions.

During the past three decades, there has been a cumulative increase in the youth population worldwide (Table 1). The bulk of this increase has been in developing nations, in which fertility rates are more than double those in developed regions.

Nature and scope of adolescent health problems

Mortality and morbidity data provide a substantial basis for measuring the extent, and for understanding the nature, of the burden of illness. The total burden of illness is not, however, comprehended through these figures exclusively[2] – it also includes the loss of potential productivity (workdays, earnings) and the years of life lost from a prospective life span. If these factors are taken into account, the burden of illness in adolescence increases greatly, and can be shown to cause important losses in human and economic resources for a nation.

In addition to the problems in the collection and reporting of adolescent health statistics already noted, there are other limitations, including: unreliability of some diagnostic categories, underreporting of certain conditions because of stigma or other social reasons, and lack of staff or facilities for data collection. Nonetheless, much of value can be learned from careful analysis of existing data.

Overall mortality rates for adolescents are relatively low (see Table 2). In the United States, however, adolescents are the only age-group for whom mortality rates are rising (3), and this is a matter for concern. Mortality rates are generally higher for males than for females (4. P. 163). Among females, complications of pregnancy, childbirth, and the puerperium are leading causes of death, especially in girls below 18 years of age (5. P. 42). Among males, accidents are the leading cause of death, followed by suicide and homicide (5. P. 41).

The morbidity data are gathered from hospitals, outpatient clinics, school health systems, and reports from physicians and other health personnel. These data are less uniform and their collection is less systematic than is the case for mortality data. Moreover, these data supply only information on adolescents who have sought help in health-care settings. Inasmuch as adolescents in both developed and developing nations are not inclined to seek medical help, the figures reported probably are a serious underestimate of the problems. Also, it is quite clear that data on psychosocial problems of adolescents are especially unreliable. There is a pressing need for epidemiologic research on health/mental health problems of adolescents, particularly in the developing nations. Ideally, surveys of adolescents should include collection of data on the health of adolescents in the community in addition to information from health facilities.

The most significant finding in health statistics worldwide with respect to adolescent health status is the extraordinary importance of behavioural factors in the leading causes of death and as contributors to the total burden of illness among the young. The relevant conditions include accidents, suicide, homicide, adolescent pregnancy, smoking, alcohol abuse, drug abuse, and other conditions related to psychosocial stress.

Impressive gains in adolescent health and a firm basis for reducing adult morbidity and mortality could be achieved by greater understanding of effective ways to change adolescents' behaviour toward promoting health and preventing

Table 2. *Principal causes of death in children and young people in 1969 and 1975*

10–14 year-olds

	USA		Central America		South America	
	Cause	%	Cause	%	Cause	%
1969						
	1	50.2	1	17.2	1	27.1
	2	13.0	5	13.9	4	8.9
	3	4.7	4	8.9	2	4.3
	4	3.7	6	4.2	6	4.2
	6	2.6	8	3.4	9	3.6
	10	25.6	10	52.4	10	51.9
	Total	100	Total	100	Total	100
1975						
	1	53.4	1	26.1	1	28.1
	2	12.0	5	9.9	4	8.3
	3	4.5	4	7.5	2	5.8
	7	3.3	6	4.8	6	4.6
	6	2.7	2	4.0	9	3.3
	10	24.1	10	47.7	10	49.9
	Total	100	Total	100	Total	100

15–19 year-olds

	USA		Central America		South America	
	Cause	%	Cause	%	Cause	%
1969						
	1	61.7	1	24.3	1	30.2
	7	6.4	4	7.1	9	5.5
	2	6.4	5	7.1	4	5.4
	10	5.1	7	4.8	2	4.9
	6	2.1	6	4.4	6	4.9
	11	18.3	11	52.3	11	49.0
	Total	100	Total	100	Total	100
1975						
	1	59.6	1	30.8	1	32.7
	7	8.7	7	8.4	7	5.7
	10	7.7	6	6.1	2	5.2
	2	5.9	4	4.9	6	5.0
	6	1.9	5	4.2	10	5.0
	11	16.2	11	45.6	11	46.4
	Total	100	Total	100	Total	100

1. Accidents
2. Malignant neoplasms
3. Congenital anomalies
4. Influenza and pneumonia
5. Enteritis and other diarrhoeal diseases
6. Cardiac diseases
7. Homicides and operations of war
8. Anaemias
9. Tuberculosis
10. Suicides
11. Other diseases

Source: Pan American Health Organization. *Condiciones de salud del niño en las Americas* (Scientific Publication No. 381). Washington, DC, Pan American Health Organization, 1979. P. 40.

disease. A range of biologic, personal, and sociocultural factors interact to influence the patterns of adolescent behaviours. The interplay of these factors will be considered in discussing the major health problems faced by adolescents and the implications for future directions in research.

Factors in adolescent health
Socio-economic

In considering the social and economic factors that affect the health of adolescents, the life-span perspective must be emphasized. Some earlier life conditions and experiences heavily influence adolescent health status. In turn, the health-related behaviours and attitudes that characterize the adolescent set patterns for adult health values, beliefs, and behaviours, for better or worse.

The initial impacts of poverty on health begin before conception. Among the poor there is greater likelihood of pregnancy and out-of-wedlock birth, and these are occurring increasingly frequently among adolescents. Among married women there is a strong relationship between poverty and completed family size: the number of births per family is much higher among the poor. Also related to poverty is the probability of less adequate prenatal care, more obstetrical complications, and early death or damage to the infants.

Accidents (Table 3), which cause significant handicap, disfigurement, disability, and death are especially frequent in adolescence. In the United States, many of the accidents among adolescents and young adults are linked with affluence and are preponderantly motor vehicle accidents, often alcohol-related (6). There is also significant mortality and morbidity among US youth from falls, drownings, burns, and other accidents. There seems to be a developmental link between risk-taking behaviour and accidents among adolescents.

Education

Education is an important factor in adolescent health, especially among girls. In developed countries, the occurrence of illegitimate, early adolescent pregnancy is positively linked to low educational status. Also, at all ages and in most societies, the least-educated mothers tend to have the largest number of children. The educational level of the mother has also been linked to health outcomes for children, independent of socioeconomic status.

In general, it is recognized that the life options of adolescents are directly related to the benefits of education.

Nutrition

Malnutrition refers to more than undernutrition: it encompasses faulty or poor nutrition in all of its aspects, which may include overnutrition or obesity and nutrient imbalances.

Table 3. *Age-specific death rates from accidents per 100 000 population by country*

Country	Year	Death rate All ages	10–14 years	15–19 years
Argentina	1970	54.9	24.1	47.7
Colombia	1975	48.0	23.6	44.6
Costa Rica	1976	42.6	14.7	31.9
Cuba	1976	35.7	19.0	34.3
Chile	1976	62.9	20.1	38.1
Dominican Republic	1975	25.5	11.1	20.0
Ecuador	1974	53.3	26.6	41.7
El Salvador	1974	47.2	24.7	40.0
Mexico	1974	60.1	27.4	54.4
Nicaragua	1976	53.8	18.0	56.0
Panama	1974	49.0	30.0	46.8
Paraguay	1976	36.4	15.7	31.0
Peru	1972	28.6	11.0	19.8
Puerto Rico	1975	35.4	15.3	32.8
USA	1976	49.1	17.7	59.2
Uruguay	1976	40.3	12.7	28.9
Venezuela	1975	59.5	23.0	51.2

Source: Pan American Health Organization. *Condiciones de salud del niño en las Americas* (Scientific Publication No. 381). Washington, DC, Pan American Health Organization, 1979. P. 48.

All forms of malnutrition exist in the United States, but their relative prevalences are not well documented. It is clear, however, that obesity is the most common form of adult malnutrition and is a major link to hypertension, myocardial infarction, and type-II diabetes. There is evidence that obesity in childhood and adolescence is predictive of adult obesity.

In Western, industrialized nations, anorexia nervosa is a prominent emotional disorder among adolescent girls. Its incidence appears to be rising over the past two decades. It is a potentially life-threatening condition in which there is self-imposed starvation. It is, however, a much more complex condition than dieting out of control: it is a serious emotional disorder that involves family relations, disturbed body image, overachievement needs, concern for control, sexuality, and, often, a prominent element of depression. It may require hospitalization for the starvation and behavioural symptoms. Treatment modalities can include medically regulated feeding, behaviour modification, antidepressant drugs, and psychotherapy. Anorexia nervosa is difficult to treat.

In Latin America, undernutrition is the major form of malnutrition (7). Protein-energy malnutrition (PEM) and iodine and iron deficiencies are major health concerns.

The growth changes in adolescence are second only to those in infancy in intensity, and we need more information on the nutritional requirements of the adolescent growth spurt. Standard measures of height and weight provide valuable data, but there is a need for reliable, rapid, non-invasive indicators for assessing nutritional status that do not require venipuncture – for example, micromethods that can use blood from a finger stick, or urinary measures.

Adolescent pregnancy

Issues of adolescent pregnancy and child-bearing were catapulted into prominence in the United States in 1976 with the publication of the Alan Guttmacher Institute's report entitled *11 million teenagers: What can be done about the epidemic of adolescent pregnancies in the United States?* (8). Since that time, the problem of adolescent fertility has continued to be high on the national agenda and received a great deal of study and intervention. Much has been documented concerning the medical, personal, social, and economic costs of too early pregnancy.

Although adolescent pregnancy is not new to Latin America, only in the recent past has it emerged as a major concern of health personnel and policymakers. The general problems are very similar to those in the United States, but there are also many specifics that differ according to the particular country, or even according to locations within a given country.

Unless countermeasures are taken, adolescent fertility in Latin America can be expected to increase substantially, because the rise is related to three factors that will have an enduring influence over the coming years. First, there is an increasing trend toward youthfulness of the overall populations of Latin American countries; the problem therefore becomes highly significant partly because of the sheer projected numbers of the population at risk. Adolescents constitute a considerably higher percentage of the population in Latin American nations than in Europe and North America. These percentages will continue to rise because the proportion of children under 15 years of age is significantly higher, at times double those of the United States. Second, there are rising rates of non-marital sexuality among those adolescents. Third, use of contraception by adolescents in Latin America is minimal and actively resisted.

The seriousness of the problem is highlighted by the fact that mortality related to childbirth is ranked as one of the five leading causes of death among women 15–19 years of age in most of the 19 countries of the Americas (4. P. 195; 5). Moreover, rising rates of venereal diseases among adolescents is a leading cause of morbidity (5. P. 52), and abortion-related deaths are significant among adolescents (4. P. 196).

Consequences of adolescent pregnancy

It is a general finding that pregnancies in young adolescents are associated with highly negative medical, psychosocial, and economic consequences for both mother and child.

Medical

Infants born to adolescent mothers, compared with mothers in their 20s, are reported to be at increased risk for prematurity, low birthweight, neural tube defects, and disproportionately high mortality (*9, 10*). Research has shown that for young pregnant adolescents (*11, 12*), the outcomes for both mother and child are not simply dependent on young age but are explained by nutritional status and by health-related behaviours such as prenatal care and use of cigarettes, alcohol, or other drugs.

Questions have been raised about physiological immaturity as an additional risk factor in the youngest adolescents, i.e. mothers aged 15 years or younger (*13–15*). Although the birth outcomes are notably worse in this age category, no definitive physiologic or anatomic changes related to maturity have been demonstrated except for a possible decrease in pelvic dimensions and the specific problem, for some, of cephalo-pelvic disproportion.

The role of nutrition is clearer. In non-obese adult women, there is a strong relationship between pregnancy weight gain and infant birthweight (*16*). Mothers of all ages who are underweight when they conceive and who gain less than 7 kg during pregnancy have a 40% risk of delivering a small for gestational age infant (*17*). When the data have been reviewed by age groups, it has been found that for adolescent mothers 10–16 years of age, babies are more growth retarded compared with children of older mothers of the same nutritional status (*18, 19*). Pregnant adolescents appear to retain nitrogen less efficiently than adult pregnant women (*20*).

These findings suggest that protein calorie intake is a crucial determinant of adolescent pregnancy outcome. Continuing undernutrition or malnutrition of adolescent mothers has been shown to produce an increasing incidence of low birthweight and foetal wastage with each subsequent pregnancy of mothers who deliver their first child in the early years of adolescence (*21*).

Repeated studies have shown that adolescent mothers, compared with adult mothers, have notably increased rates of toxaemia (*22, 23*). They also have increased incidences of amniotic fluid infections, placental abruptions, and prolonged or precipitous labours. Implications of these all too frequent complications of pregnancy for the later health of the adolescent are as yet unknown.

Psychosocial

When adolescent students become pregnant, this often means that their schooling will be interrupted or halted, and the life options of the young person will be significantly reduced. In the United States this is usually due to voluntary dropping out of school. In many Latin American countries, the pregnant adolescent is required to leave school. Unemployment or work at only menial, low-paying jobs throughout adult life then becomes much more likely. In any case, the educational and psychological growth of the young adolescent is usually curtailed.

A substantial majority of adolescent mothers are unmarried and live in unstable situations of transient common-law unions, under crowded conditions with the family of origin, or isolated in single-parent households. Young adolescent mothers are likely to have children in rapid succession and a larger completed family size than those who begin child-bearing in adulthood. All of these are situations of great psychosocial stress for the mother and her child, or children.

Children of adolescent mothers tend to show higher percentages of developmental, behavioural, and cognitive difficulties than children of older mothers. It is generally believed that these negative outcomes represent an interactive phenomenon. Many of the children of adolescent mothers have perinatal complications that are handicapping to varying degrees. A significant number of them may not have demonstrable neurological or physiological deficits, but are irritable or difficult children (24). It has been suggested that this difficult temperament may be a risk factor for later behavioural difficulty (25) because of mother–child interaction problems.

The developmental outcome for the child depends not only on health status at birth but also on the subsequent care-taking environment. Significant socioenvironmental factors may include poor nutrition, inadequate stimulation, inappropriate expectations (26), and parental rejection. Adolescent mothers have been shown to spend less time with their infants and to engage in less verbal interaction with them. When there are child-rearing supports from the adolescent's extended family, the developmental outcome for the infant is enhanced (27–29).

Rise in sexual activity

The secular trend toward earlier menarche that has occurred over the past 100 years because of improved health and nutrition in affluent nations means that sexual and reproductive readiness is now occurring at unusually low ages (30). At the same time, induction into adult roles has been postponed to uncommonly high ages. Adolescents have been expected to remain sexually abstinent during this lengthy period. Traditionally, there have been strong moral and religious constraints on engaging in adolescent and premarital sexual activity.

In the United States, the decade from 1970 to 1980 saw a sharp rise in adolescent and premarital sexual activity. For example, the median age of initiation of activity has dropped from 18 to 16 years, and rates of sexual activity for girls under 16 are ten times higher than they were in the Kinsey survey of 1953 (31, 32). These dramatic changes reflect, in part, major social changes, including in the roles of women, permissive sexual attitudes, legalization of abortion, and availability of contraceptives. There is also a heightened media emphasis on youthfulness and sexuality. Issues associated with adolescent sexuality have become particularly acute in the United States, but there is now growing concern in other developed countries and in developing nations as well.

It has become increasingly clear that in developing nations the phenomena of urbanization, migration to cities, and social and cultural dislocation are affecting adolescents. They are experiencing major social changes in a context in which there is often a breakdown of traditional family patterns and cultural constraints.

Attitudes toward contraception
In the United States, following extensive educational campaigns linked with easy availability of contraceptives, adult women, married women of all ages, and older adolescents quite commonly practise reliable contraception. The youngest adolescents are the ones most likely not to use contraceptives; they have been unresponsive to the approaches that have been successful with older women.

In 1973, the Supreme Court made abortion a legal option for all women in the United States. The trend in the abortion rate was steadily upward until 1979, when it levelled off. In 1983, evidence of a decline was noted that appeared to reflect a decrease in pregnancy rate. The data showed that of the approximately one million pregnant adolescents, just over 400 000 obtained abortions. Use of abortion by adolescents remains controversial despite its legal status because it raises significant, unresolved issues about the appropriate and possibly conflicting relationships between the rights and the interests of the individual adolescent, her family, and the state.

Although abortion for the very youngest teenagers (15 years or younger) remains a special issue, there are no data that would either support or refute such age restrictions. No evidence is available concerning the capacity of adolescents to make such decisions or on psychological consequences of abortion.

Several states have, in recent years, passed laws that restrict minors' access to abortion services without parental consent or that limit judicial bypass of such consent. Research has not documented that legally required parental involvement helps teenage girls cope better with their choice to terminate a pregnancy. There is no evidence that parental involvement reduces the probability of subsequent unwanted pregnancies or that it served any purpose beyond ensuring that parents are informed of the intentions of their pregnant daughter. There is, however, growing evidence that statutes on parental consent do cause teenagers to delay their abortions, if for no other reason than that they must undergo the *de facto* waiting period associated with finding a lawyer and gaining access to the courts. These delays may increase the health risks involved if they result in postponements until the second trimester of pregnancy. There is also increasing evidence that many adolescents in states with these statutes are travelling to nearby states to obtain services rather than go through the judicial bypass procedure. But it is not currently known whether such statutes are causing an increase in unwanted births to teenagers. Research is needed on all of these difficult issues.

The question has been raised of whether or not abortion becomes a form of birth control when it is available. Although it is clear that adolescent girls in the early phase of sexual activity often do not practice contraception regularly, there is evidence that abortion is not chosen in preference to abstinence or contraception as a means of avoiding unwanted child-bearing. Repeated abortions do occur among teenagers as well as among adult women. Nevertheless, concern that the availability of abortion services will lead to higher rates of teenage sexual activity and pregnancy and less reliance on contraception is not supported by the available research. Adolescents who have had abortions are, in fact, less likely to experience another pregnancy within two years than are those who have given birth.

Most abortions occur during the first trimester of pregnancy and therefore carry little risk of medical complications when they are performed by qualified professionals in appropriately equipped settings. Although the health risks are somewhat greater for second-trimester abortions, those risks are minimized if the abortion is performed under appropriate conditions. In general, the health risks associated with an early, legal abortion are no greater for adolescents than for adult women; in most cases, they are lower. Across all ages, abortion poses significantly fewer risks than those associated with pregnancy and childbirth. Public health experts estimate that the replacement of unintended births and illegal abortions by legal abortions has averted as many as 1500 pregnancy-related deaths among American women (including teenagers) and life-threatening complications in the tens of thousands.

In many Latin American countries, abortion is illegal, and sex education and availability of contraceptives are often taboo. Negative governmental, religious, and sociocultural attitudes are a major barrier to use of contraceptives by adolescents. Despite growing concern about and recognition of teenage pregnancy as a problem, there is great reluctance, even aversion, to giving legitimacy to instruction about, and the distribution of, contraceptives.

Use and abuse of tobacco, alcohol, and other drugs

The use of tobacco and alcohol is an example of behaviour that is widely prohibited to adolescents, but socially acceptable and legal for adults. When this is the case, such substances have an attraction for many adolescents as badges of adult status, and there is a strong temptation to experiment with them and, for a significant number, to engage in their regular use at an early age. For these young people such usage may variously serve as a symbol of independence, of rebellion against conventional standards, and/or of virility.

At a time when many illegal drugs are readily available – marijuana and hashish,

LSD, amphetamines, tranquilizers, cocaine, and heroin – adults are often more comfortable when adolescents choose to use the legal substances with which the older generations are familiar. Therefore, some adults encourage adolescents in the use of alcohol and tobacco in the hope of deterring them from using illegal drugs that are perceived as more threatening.

There are other reasons for tobacco and alcohol use, differing from country to country, some cultural, and others related to economic exploitation of affluent youth; they have led to widespread and increasing adolescent use of tobacco, alcohol, and other drugs everywhere. The effects are reflected in morbidity and mortality not only during adolescence, but throughout the users' lives.

Tobacco

Heavy, long-term use of tobacco is well known to be associated with lung cancer. Although less emphasis has been given them, there are other major health effects as well – e.g. chronic bronchitis, emphysema, coronary disease, other cancers, and harmful effects on the developing foetus that result in lowered birthweight if pregnant women smoke (33, 34). At one time smoking was preponderantly a male habit; but over the past decade, particularly in urban, industrialized cultures, there has been a steep increase in smoking by women and adolescent girls (35). The risks of smoking during pregnancy now assume great importance.

Of all the major risk factors for serious illness, disability, and premature death, smoking is the most important preventable one (36). Prevention programmes should be targeted toward children and adolescents. Smoking is a habit that has extraordinary tenacity, and is often considered to be an addiction. There are reports that it is particularly difficult for women to quit smoking (37). Therefore, efforts aimed at helping adults to quit smoking are more likely to be difficult and less fruitful than programmes aimed at persuading young people not to smoke.

Data on smoking are carefully monitored in the United States, and the figures indicate that about 4000 youngsters start smoking each day (38). It is clear that when smoking goes beyond the most casual experimentation, there is a very high risk of escalation to regular use.

Although the long-term consequences of smoking are devastating and the overall burden of illness is very high, adolescents fail to appreciate the true gravity of the problem. Developmentally they have cognitive limitations that lead them to think only in terms of the current situation, and they find it very difficult to take a long-range view. Hence, the eventual, negative effects have no reality for them, and the immediate pleasure and gratification have great appeal.

One of the important factors in the initiation of smoking is peer influence. In recruiting others to the use of tobacco, peers often apply social pressure, offer role models, and make supplies of tobacco and other substances available. Adolescents are particularly sensitive to peer influences and are strongly inclined to respond to them. The use of peer influence has proved to be a promising research approach to the prevention of smoking – a subject that will be discussed further under research opportunities.

Alcohol and other drugs

Alcohol use is virtually universal everywhere in the world, and is, at the same time, the single largest contributor to morbidity and mortality. There are extraordinarily high personal costs in terms of depression, family disruption, violence, psychosis, physical disorders, accident proneness, and the occurrence of abnormalities in children born to alcohol-using mothers.

Adolescents, particularly young adolescents, are an important high-risk group. Drinking patterns in developed nations have changed markedly over the past decade; a very high proportion of adolescents have their initial drinking experience earlier, they drink in large quantities, and they report more frequent intoxication. Girls still drink less than boys, but their use of alcohol is increasing at a faster rate. They are tending to catch up and narrow the gap between male and female drinking patterns (*39, 40*). The data are comparable with those for smoking.

Unlike tobacco, alcohol and illicit drugs are mind-altering substances. The effects of such mind-altering substances on the still-developing brain tissues of young adolescents have not been fully elucidated, but it seems probable that this is another reason for special concern with regard to the youngest adolescents, and an area for research priority.

Apart from the direct effects on the brain, habitual use of mind-altering substances poses developmental risks for young adolescents. Instead of meeting the appropriate developmental tasks and challenges, habitual users of these substances often withdraw from transiently difficult, but ultimately growth-promoting, experiences and, instead, learn to cope with difficulties through chemical dependency. There is a resultant void in needed developmental learning and in acquisition of the skills necessary to be effective adults.

When young people can be persuaded to give up their drug dependencies, the tasks of re-educating and rehabilitating them are formidable. The drug use has often caused school failure, legal difficulties, and alienation of family and friends. There are deep feelings of failure and inferiority to be overcome. As with smoking, there are compelling reasons to try to prevent, or at least postpone, the use of these powerful substances by adolescents.

A problem-behaviour perspective

Health-damaging behaviour in adolescents tends to include more than one type of problem, and a problem-behaviour perspective thus seems indicated (*41*). This perspective assumes that: (1) health behaviour is functional and has meaning for the adolescent; (2) the meaning is related to the person's developmental status; (3)

the meaning is learned through social experience; (4) that experience is patterned, that is, it is non-random and non-arbitrary and reflects the societal influences to which the adolescent is exposed in terms of the norms, values, and sanctions of a given culture. As a result, not only do problem or health-damaging behaviours tend to be concurrent but the practice of one behaviour, such as smoking or alcohol use, appears to be associated with the likelihood of initiating the practice of another. For example, in the Bogolusa Health Study (42), it was found that young girls who smoked were much more likely to be involved also in sexual activity. This does not imply that one behaviour leads to, or causes, the other, but rather that the same influences and motivations underlie the various problem behaviours.

Collectively, these influences and motivations can be termed *risk factors* for problem behaviours. The risks can be divided into three categories: personal or personality factors, social or interpersonal factors, and cultural of environmental factors. The degree of influence of these factors will vary from culture to culture. Personal factors include an emphasis on unconventionality, rebelliousness, high risk-taking, low value on achievement, and high value on autonomy. Social or interpersonal factors include alienation from parents, considerable influence of peers involved in problem behaviours, and little involvement in religious activities. Cultural factors include low social controls, disorganized environment, permissive values, media pressures for smoking, drinking, and sexual indulgence, and a strong 'youth culture'.

This formulation suggests certain implications for research and promising directions for interventions in dealing with these serious problems of adolescents. The results of controlled studies on programmes to prevent smoking, for example, have shown that the onset of smoking can be delayed for at least two years. It is too soon to know whether, for many young people, the use of tobacco can be completely prevented by these social learning strategies.

The mental health of adolescents

The US President's Commission on Mental Health (43) listed adolescents among the groups with major unmet mental health needs in the United States. Suicide among adolescents is a vivid indicator of adolescent depression; it is the third leading cause of death among 15–19 year-olds. In the United States, suicides have shown a 40% increase since 1970 (Table 4). Some Latin American nations have adolescent suicide rates even higher than those in the United States (Table 5). Moreover, it is estimated that for every actual suicide, there are 100 attempted suicides.

This is a major problem about which very little is known. It is only within the past few years that depression has been recognized as a serious mental disorder among children and youth. The extent and nature of the problem now demand major research attention.

Table 4. *Suicide rates per 100 000 population among 15–19-year-olds in the United States, 1965–75*

	1965	1970	1971	1972	1973	1974	1975
Both sexes	4.0	5.9	6.5	6.9	7.0	7.2	7.6
White males	6.3	9.4	10.3	11.1	11.4	11.9	13.0
Other males	5.2	5.4	6.8	9.5	6.8	6.2	7.0
White females	1.8	2.9	3.0	2.7	3.2	3.3	3.1
Other females	2.4	2.9	3.6	3.4	2.7	2.8	2.1

Source: US Secretary of Health, Education and Welfare. *Health United States, 1976–1977* (Publication No. (HRA) 77-1232). Washington, DC, 1977, as cited in *Condiciones de salud del niño en las Americas* (Scientific Publication No. 381). Washington, DC, Pan American Health Organization, 1979. P. 46.

There are other important, although less dramatic, symptoms of the costs of psychosocial stress in adolescents. Psychosomatic disorders are prominent in this age group.

Violence is a serious health concern for adolescents – males, in particular. In the United States this is dramatically indicated by the fact that homicide is one of the three leading causes of death among youth. In addition to this tragic statistic, there is school violence, which often makes urban schools a dangerous place for teachers and students; and there are street crime and violence within the family. Very often adolescents are victims of violence and abuse both within the home and on the streets. The largest single source of the runaways and the 'emancipated youths' who flock to, and are exploited in, large cities are boys and girls who are fleeing family violence, physical and/or sexual abuse.

Currently these problems are identified chiefly with minority and disadvantaged youth in inner cities, and seem to relate to health and mental health problems of urbanization, structural unemployment, poverty, failures of schooling, and lack of legitimate avenues for the adolescent energy, and normative risk-taking, needed to assert mastery. Even with improvements in national economies, the unemployment of youth is likely to persist as a long-term feature of industrialized nations.

Serious thought must be given to means by which the energies and aspirations of youth can be harnessed in ways that promote self-discipline, self-respect, and earned esteem through positive contributions to society. New social inventions or institutions are needed to foster systematic, constructive activity during the extended years of older adolescence that industrialized societies confer upon their youth. Suggestions along these lines are now being put forward in the United States (45) for consideration by policymakers. For example, a national youth service for adolescents that would be a form of domestic Peace Corps is being studied as

Table 5. *Suicide deaths per 100 000 population for selected age groups for selected countries, 1976 or the most recent year*

Country	Year	Suicide death rate		
		All ages	10–14 years	15–19 years
Argentina	1970	9.7	1.3	8.4
Colombia	1975	3.6	0.8	7.5
Costa Rica	1976	5.7	0.3	5.9
Cuba	1976	17.6	3.9	24.3
Chile	1976	5.6	1.4	6.2
Dominican Republic	1975	3.3	1.2	5.3
Ecuador	1974	2.6	—	4.8
El Salvador	1974	10.8	—	26.7
Mexico	1974	2.1	—	4.0
Nicaragua	1976	0.6	—	1.2
Panama	1974	3.0	—	3.6
Paraguay	1976	3.5	0.5	6.2
Peru	1972	1.8	—	3.2
Puerto Rico	1975	7.7	1.3	2.4
USA	1976	12.5	0.8	7.4
Uruguay	1976	10.9	1.6	7.7
Venezuela	1975	5.0	0.9	5.8

Source: Pan American Health Organization, *Condiciones de salud del niño en las Americas.* Washington, DC, Pan American Health Organization, 1979. p. 45

one approach. Schools are experimenting with a variety of ways in which adolescents can perform supervised work in the community with pre-schoolers or the elderly; and the business community is trying out a number of interventions that will link schools with the work world.

There is a growing societal consensus that serious attention must be paid to meeting the needs of at-risk youth as an important aspect of bettering society as a whole by improving the health, education, and well-being of its future workers, parents, and citizens.

Priorities and opportunities in future research

Current demographic trends and emerging patterns of social change underscore the importance of heightened concern by policymakers and the health-care establishment for the health and well-being of the adolescent sector of our populations. The number of adolescents is large and is increasing worldwide. There are continuing pressures toward industrialization and urbanization in developing countries that will have consequences for adolescent health in multiple ways.

Experience in industrialized nations suggests that rapid social change, breakdown of family supports, and prolongation of adolescence have been associated with an exacerbation of adolescent problems and an increase in health-damaging behaviours.

The training of medical professionals and health-care workers who are involved in primary care should give appropriate emphasis to adolescent health needs and should include substantial information on adolescent physical and psychosocial development. Health personnel should be trained to collaborate effectively with workers who are in contact with adolescents in other sectors, such as education, social services, and youth workers who interact with out-of-school adolescents. New and relevant knowledge and findings of research should be systematically disseminated to medical schools and training centres.

In many nations there are very few data on which to base the planning to meet adolescent health needs. National health statistical systems, when they exist, tend to report adolescent data for a single age-group, commonly 15–19 years. Current knowledge suggests that this is inadequate on two counts. First, the age-range is too narrow, for significant problems are occurring in younger adolescents. The age-range should extend down to at least 12 years of age; and in urban, industrial areas, monitoring tobacco, alcohol, and drug abuse must begin at 10 years of age. Second, there are clear indications of great differences in morbidity and health risks across the 12–20 year age span. Two age groupings are highly useful: 12–16 years and 17–20 years. For example, the youngest adolescents are at very high risk for morbidity and mortality in relation to pregnancy, whereas 18- and 19-year-olds may represent the optimum period for childbirth and are at low medical risk.

It is also important to break down reported data for out-of-school and in-school adolescents. The magnitude of the non-student youth populations is great in developing nations. Many of these young people migrate to urban areas, and their health status is not known. It can be assumed that their health problems will be considerable. Establishing preventive and treatment services that can reach this population presents greater challenges.

Studies of new uses for established health facilities are needed. Several unintegrated types of services deal in one way or another with adolescent health needs: general health, maternal and child health, school health, military and occupational health (including medical examination for vocational guidance), family-planning, and prevention. Primary-care health workers should be aware of all of these opportunities for reaching adolescents.

Research is needed on ways in which more comprehensive care can be given to adolescents within a particular health context. For example, the integration into primary-care facilities of clinics for family planning for sexually active teenagers would permit this problem to be dealt with regardless of the presenting symptoms that bring the adolescent to the health centre.

Adolescents tend not to seek medical care. When in contact with health clinics, they are resistant to services unless there is assurance of confidentiality, understanding, and a non-judgmental attitude toward them. Studies of how to improve the motivation of adolescents to seek care and how to increase compliance with regard to the psychosocial aspects of health care are greatly needed.

Efforts to make effective use of community and voluntary resources should be fostered. Important health-education activities and some forms of health services can be developed by neighbourhood and community workers. Adolescents themselves can play a significant role in such activities. More research is needed on adolescent and general community participation in health activities.

Depending on the country, the schools constitute a more or less sizable percentage of adolescents readily accessible to health-care and -education efforts. Many learning and school discipline problems have significant areas of medical concern. Research is needed on new ways of delivering school health services so that they are preventive and comprehensive. The schools may offer the single best opportunity to reach and meet the health needs of adolescents who are fortunate enough to be students.

In the United States, schools have been utilized for important research on the prevention of smoking of tobacco by adolescents. Using principles of social learning and knowledge of adolescent development, a number of investigators have studied the efficacy of a combined educational and peer-mediated approach. Following a presentation of complete information on the health hazards of smoking and the short-term effects on athletic fitness and personal attractiveness, adolescents are involved in programmes designed to use peer pressure in positive ways to foster a commitment to non-smoking and to actively develop strategies to counteract pressures to smoke that may be exerted by other peers, the media, or adults. Successful programmes have also used peer counseling and role-playing techniques (46–48).

Although the programmes described have been limited to tobacco, there are good reasons to believe that the same approaches can and should be used in tandem to mount preventive interventions against alcohol and substance abuse. Success in such efforts would represent a significant gain.

Research is greatly needed with regard to developmentally appropriate and culturally relevant educational efforts regarding substance abuse. In the United States much of the drug education has been ineffective or counterproductive. There is still a great deal to be learned about linking adolescent cognitive level, motivational structures, and active learning techniques with informational content in ways that can catch and hold adolescents' attention and teach them what they need to know to avoid harmful practices and promote health.

Notes

1. A. Pusey, Behaviours of juveniles among free-living chimpanzee. Unpublished doctoral thesis, Stanford University, 1977.
2. D. Rice, The current burden of illness in the United States. Plenary address at the Institute of Medicine, National Academy of Sciences, Washington, DC, 27 October 1987.

References

1. Denney, R. American youth today. *Daedalus*, Winter, pp. 124–44 (1962).
2. Wyshak, G., & Frisch, R. E. Evidence for a secular trend in the age of menarche. *New England Journal of Medicine*, **306**, 1033–35 (1982).
3. US Department of Health and Human Services. Death rates from selected causes by age, race, sex (Tables 15–22). In *Health: United States 1981*. Washington, DC, US Government Printing Office, 1981. Pp. 120–42.
4. Pan American Health Organization. *Health conditions in the Americas, 1973–1976* (Scientific Publication No. 364). Washington, DC, Pan American Health Organization, 1978.
5. Pan American Health Organization. *Condiciones de salud del niño en las Americas* (Scientific Publication No. 381). Washington, DC, Pan American Health Organization, 1979.
6. Kovar, M. G. Adolescent health status and health-related behaviour. In *Adolescent behaviour and health. A conference summary*. Washington, DC, National Academy of Sciences, 1978.
7. Pollitt, E. *Poverty and malnutrition in Latin America*. New York, Praeger, 1980. P. 39.
8. Alan Guttmacher Institute. *11 million teenagers: What can be done about the epidemic of adolescent pregnancies in the United States?* New York, Planned Parenthood Federation of America, 1976.
9. Baldwin, W., & Cain, V. S. The children of teenage parents. *Family Planning Perspectives*, **12** (January/February), 34–43 (1980).
10. Mermitt, J., Lawrence, R., & Naeye, R. The infants of adolescent mothers. *Pediatric Annals*, **9**, 32–46 (1980).
11. Hingson, S., Alpert, J., Day, N., Dooling, E., Kayne, H., Morelock, S., Oppenheimer, E., Rosett, H., Weiner, L., & Zuckerman, B. Effects of maternal drinking, smoking and psychoactive drug use on fetal development. *Pediatrics*, **70**, 539–46 (1982).
12. Naeye, R. L. Teenaged and pre-teenaged pregnancies: Consequences of the fetal-maternal competition for nutrients. *Pediatrics*, **67**, 146–40 (1981).
13. Zlatnick, F. J., & Bermeister, C. F. Low 'gynecologic age': An obstetric risk factor. *American Journal of Obstetrics and Gynecology*, **128**, 183–86 (1977).
14. Hollingsworth, D. R., & Kotchen, J. M. Gynecologic age and its relation to neonatal outcome. *Birth Defects*, **17** (3), 91–105 (1981).

15. Morrison, J. H. Primiparas under age fourteen. *American Journal of Obstetrics and Gynecology*, **84**, 442–48 (1962).
16. Rosso, P., & Cramoy, C. Nutrition and pregnancy. In M. Winick (Ed.), *Nutrition: Pre- and post-natal development*. New York, Plenum, 1979. Pp. 133–228.
17. Rosso, P. Pre-natal nutrition and fetal growth development. *Pediatric Annals*, **10** (11), 21–32 (1981).
18. Naeye, R. L. Nutritional/non-nutritional interactions that affect the outcome of pregnancy. *American Journal of Clinical Nutrition*, **34** (April), Suppl., pp. 727–31 (1981).
19. Morse, E. G., Clarke, R. P., Merrow, S. B., & Thilbault, B. E. Comparison of the nutritional status of pregnant adolescents with adult pregnant women: Anthropometric and dietary findings. *American Journal of Clinical Nutrition*, **28** (December), 1422–28 (1975).
20. King, J. C., Calloway, D. H., & Margen, S. Nitrogen retention, total body K, and weight gain in teenage pregnant girls. *Journal of Nutrition*, **103**, 772–78 (1973).
21. Jekel, J., Harrison, J., Bancroft, D., Tyler, N., & Klerman, L. A comparison of health of index and subsequent babies born to school-age mothers. *American Journal of Public Health*, **65**, 370–74 (1975).
22. Israel, S. L., & Woutersz, T. B. Teenage obstetrics. *American Journal of Obstetrics*, **85**, 659–68 (1963).
23. Hutchins, F. L., Jr., Kendal, N., & Rubino, J. Experience with teenage pregnancy. *Journal of the American College of Obstetrics and Gynecology*, **54** (1), 1–5 (1979).
24. Rothenberg, B., & Varga, P. The relationship between age of mother and child health and development. *American Journal of Public Health*, **81**, 810–21 (1981).
25. Porter, R., & Collins, G. M. (Eds.) *Temperamental differences in infants and young children* (Ciba Foundation Symposium 89). London, Pittman, 1982.
26. Oppel, W., & Royston, A. Teenage births: Some social, psychological, and physical sequelae. *American Journal of Public Health*, **61**, 751–56 (1971).
27. Hamburg, B. Teenagers as parents: Developmental issues in teenage pregnancy. In E. Purcell (Ed.), *Psychopathology of children and youth*. New York, Josiah Macy, Jr., Foundation, 1980. Pp. 299–321.
28. Furstenberg, F. F. *Unplanned parenthood: The social consequences of teenage childbearing*. New York, Macmillan, 1976.
29. Zuckerman, B., Winsmore, G., & Alpert, J. A study of attitudes and support systems of inner city adolescent mothers. *Journal of Pediatrics*, **95**, 122–25 (1979).
30. Tanner, J. M. *Growth at adolescence* (2nd ed.). London, Blackwell, 1962. Pp. 94–143.
31. Vener, A. M., Steward, C. S., & Hager, D. L. The sexual behaviour of adolescents in Middle America: Generational and American-British comparisons. *Journal of Marriage and the Family*, **34**, 693–705 (1972).
32. Kinsey, A., Pomeroy, W., & Gebhard, P. H. *Sexual behaviour in the human female*. Philadelphia, Saunders, 1953.

33. Adams, E. E. Mortality. In *Smoking and health: A report of the Surgeon-General* (DHEW Pub. No. 79-50066). Washington, DC, US Government Printing Office, 1979. Chap. 1, pp. 1–47.

34. Hasselmeyer, E. G., Meyer, M. B., Catz, C., & Longo, L. D. Pregnancy and infant health. In *Smoking and health: A report of the Surgeon-General* (DHEW Pub. No. 79-50066). Washington, DC, US Government Printing Office, 1979. Chap. 8, pp. 2–93.

35. Bachman, J. G., Johnston, L. D., & O'Malley, P. M. Smoking, drinking, and drug use among American high school students: Correlates and trends, 1975–1979. *American Journal of Public Health*, **71**, 59–69 (1981).

36. US Department of Health, Education and Welfare. Smoking and health: Special objectives. In *Promoting health/preventing disease: Objectives for the nation* (Report of a conference in Atlanta, GA, August 1979). Reprinted by the Department of Health and Human Services. Washington, DC, US Government Printing Office, 1984. Pp. 61–63.

37. Jarvik, M. Biological influences on cigarette smoking. In *Smoking and health: A report of the Surgeon-General* (DHEW Pub. No. 79-50066). Washington, DC, US Government Printing Office, 1979. Chap. 15, pp. 1–40.

38. Johnston, L. D., Bachman, J. G., & O'Malley, P. M. Cigarettes. In *Student drug use in America, 1975–1981* (National Institute of Drug Abuse). Washington, DC, US Government Printing Office, 1981.

39. Fishburne, P. M., & Cisin, I. *National survey on drug abuse: Main findings 1979* National Institute of Drug Abuse (DHHS Pub. No. 80–976). Washington, DC, US Government Printing Office, 1980.

40. Johnston, L. D., Bachman, J. G., & O'Malley, P. M. Alcohol. In *Student drug use in America, 1975–1981* (National Institute of Drug Abuse). Washington, DC, US Government Printing Office, 1981.

41. Jessor, R., & Jessor, S. L. *Problem behaviour and psychosocial development*. New York, Academic Press, 1977.

42. Hunter, S. M., Webber, L. S., & Berenson, G. S. Cigarette smoking and tobacco usage behaviour in children and adolescents: Bogolusa Heart Study. *Preventative Medicine*, **9**, 701–712 (1980).

43. President's Commission on Mental Health. *The mental health of infants, children and adolescents* (Task Panel reports submitted to the President's Commission on Mental Health) (DHHS Publ No. 0403000-000392-4). Washington, DC, US Government Printing Office, 1978. Vol. 3, Appendix, pp. 661–729.

44. Harburg, E., Erfurt, J. C., & Chape, C. Socioecological stressor areas and black-white blood pressure: Detroit. *Journal of Chronic Diseases*, **26**, 595–611 (1976).

45. The States' Excellence in Education Commission. *Who's looking out for at-risk youth*. Flint, MI, The Charles Stewart Mott Foundation, 1985.

46. Evans, R. I. Smoking in children and adolescents: Psychosocial determinants and preventive strategies. In *Smoking and health: A report of the Surgeon-General* (DHEW Pub. No. 79-50066). Washington, DC, US Government Printing Office, 1979. Chap. 17, pp. 1–30.

47. Perry, C. L., & Murray, D. M. Enhancing the transition years: The challenge of adolescent health promotion. *Journal of School Health,* **52**, 307–311 (1982).

48. Botvin, G. J. Broadening the focus of smoking prevention strategies. In T. J. Coates, A. C. Petersen, & C. L. Perry (Eds.), *Promoting adolescent health: A Dialog on research and practice.* New York, Academic Press, 1982. Pp. 137–48.

6

Social networks and mental disorder (with special reference to the elderly)

Heinz Häfner & Rainer Welz

In the preservation of mental health, supportive social networks such as family, neighbours, and friends enjoy increasing importance. The network of personal relationships plays a decisive part in the growth of identity, transmission of social norms and attitudes, decision making, and coping with crises and stressful life events.

Essential elements of the social support concept can already be found in the work of E. Durkheim (1), who, 90 years ago, examined the influence of societal factors on suicide frequencies. It is these studies that gave rise to the theory of social disintegration. Durkheim explained the integrating function of groups by basically psychological concepts. He noted that if a group is characterized by a low degree of integration, the individual withdraws from the social life of that group and gives precedence to his own goals rather than in those of the group. This leads to a disintegration of the normative nexus of the group and to a reduction in the number of opportunities for effective support. Since Durkheim's time, the concept of 'social isolation' rather than his original concept of 'social disintegration' has become increasingly important in research on social and psychological conditions of mental health.

Faris & Dunham (2) found high incidences of certain categories of mental disorders in areas of Chicago with a high proportion of single-person households. We were able to confirm these findings in the German industrial city of Mannheim in 1965 (3). Sainsbury (4), in London, found a high correlation between suicide rate and the proportion of persons living alone or in communal housing, such as homes for the elderly. Epidemiological research on schizophrenia, depression, and mental illness in old age has consistently revealed higher rates in areas with high rates

Professor Dr Häfner is Director of the Zentralinstitut für Seelische Gesundheit, P.O. Box 5970, D-6800 Mannheim, FRG. Dr Welz, who was formerly with the same institute, is now with the Department of Medical Psychology, University of Göttingen, Humboldt-Allee, 3 FRG.

of one-person households. Nevertheless, the aggregate area characteristic 'rate of one-person households' is only one indicator; it alone does not prove a direct association between social isolation and risk of mental illness.

In recent years, investigation of social isolation as a factor influencing the genesis, course, and outcome of mental disorders has given way to network analysis (first undertaken by E. Bott (5) in an investigation of working-class families in London) as a paradigm in psychiatric epidemiology. In such an analysis priority is given to examination of the effects relationships within the personal network and the systems of social support have on the risk of falling ill, on the course of illness, and on coping with physical and mental disorders.

The structure of social networks

Networks evolve from social interactions that individuals have with other individuals according to their interests and ties. They represent systems of transactions characterized by exchange of information, wielding of authority, exertion of social influence, coordination of activities, and mobilization of social support.

There are considerable quantitative differences in the structures of social networks of the population in general and those of persons suffering from mental disorders. In comparison with the general population, in which the average network of primary contacts includes 40 to 45 persons, of whom 6 to 10 are very close friends or relatives (6), people suffering from mental disorders have considerably more limited networks. According to Pattison, Francisco, & Wood (7), the networks of the mentally ill were found to consist of 10 to 12 people, some of whom were idealized, lived far away, or were already dead. Moreover, among these, dependency relationships frequently prevailed (7, 8).

Welz, Veill, & Häfner (59) found quantitatively smaller social networks among people who had attempted suicide. The differences were significant in terms of the number of both friends and acquaintances and relatives and family members with whom these people maintained regular contacts, and the findings were independent of whether the subjects lived in one-person households or with partners. Though the controls had contacts with relatives and family members about as rarely as the subjects who had attempted suicide, their circle of friends and acquaintances was twice as large.

The functions of social networks

Among the various benefits of membership in a social group, the social support and emotional ties it affords is of special importance for coping with stressful life events and the preservation of mental health.

Nuckolls, Cassel, & Kaplan (9) found complications of pregnancy to be less frequent among women with sufficient social support compared with a group of

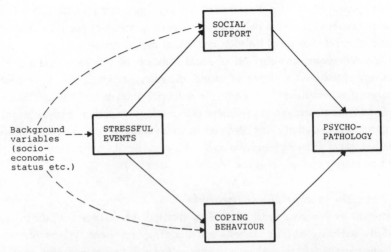

Fig. 1. The relationship between social environment and psychiatric disorders.

women with inadequate social-support resources. Among men who had become jobless, Cobb (*10*) showed depression scores to co-vary with the amount of social support provided by friends and family members.

The protective effect of social support against the risk of mental illness has been demonstrated by two studies conducted in Australia (*11, 12*). Andrews and co-workers (*11*), who conducted a field study in Melbourne, found that 80% of the people who in stressful life events could rely on the help and support of their relatives, friends, and neighbours showed no signs, or only slight signs, of mental disorder, compared with 70% of those with no such support. A further comparison of the two extreme groups makes the difference still clearer: those with few stressful life events and adequate personal and social-support resources had a morbidity rate for neurotic disorders of 12.8%, whereas subjects exposed to a large number of stressors who had inadequate personal and social-support resources had a rate of 43.3%. Similar findings were achieved by Henderson and colleagues (*12*) in Canberra. Their aim was to prove that, irrespective of stressful life events, a limited or inadequate number of social relationships correlates with a greater risk for mental disorder. According to these investigators, the morbidity risk was highest for women with limited social integration and a heavy burden of stressful life events. In comparison, women with numerous stressful life events, but whose social integration was good and whose interpersonal relationships were adequate, were only half so prone to mental illness.

With regard to depressive illness (*13, 14*), the diffusely and indistinctly defined minor mental disorders (*15, 16*), and physical diseases (*17*), social support has been shown to have a mitigating (buffering) effect in stressful life events. The amount of the social support received thus constitutes an intervening variable and can, in addition to personal coping styles, be regarded as an important resource in handling stress (see Figure 1).

Stressful life events, social networks, and mental disorder in old age
The percentage of old and very old people in the world population has been constantly rising. The proportion of people over 65 years of age in the population is expected to rise by 57.7% from 1980 to 2000, and will presumably have tripled by 2025 (*18*). Even in countries where this process is less advanced, elderly people are a very vulnerable group. Because of their increasing need for support and their great vulnerability, this group seems to provide a good illustration of the importance of social networks for prevention and rehabilitation of mental disorders.

In view of the current tendency in our society for elderly people to be ousted from working life and family, old age is often accompanied by a high frequency of stressful life events, which often lead to drastic changes in elderly people's living conditions and life-styles. Examples are the death of close relatives and of friends and acquaintances and the subsequent shrinking of the network of social relationships, plus retirement, which may lead to a loss of opportunities for extrafamilial activity – even, in some cases, to a loss of sense of purpose in life. These may be joined by a loss of status, a considerable deterioration in the person's economic situation, even to the point of poverty, and, last but not least, chronic ill-health, frailty, and loss of the ability to care for oneself, resulting, eventually, in institutionalization.

The few studies conducted thus far among elderly people have focused on the effects of the loss of close relatives. One consistent finding of these studies is that the widowed have an elevated risk for depression. The research findings reported from the United States that the health and mortality risks associated with the loss of one's partner are less grave in old age compared with earlier phases of life (*19, 20*) seem to point to cultural factors. But elderly people may be better prepared for losing their partners since they perhaps reckon with it and have more often experienced it in their personal environments (*21*). This assumption may also be of importance for the differing risks associated with retirement or unemployment in the earlier phases of life (*22*).

Although elderly people may show greater psychological resistance in connection with retirement or loss of close relatives, there is no doubt that there are areas in which they exhibit greater vulnerability than younger people when confronted with certain life events. One example is a change in residence in advanced age, or institutionalization, which means loss of a familiar, ordered pattern of life and relationships. The consequence may be psycho-organic syndromes and confusional states in the elderly people concerned (*23*). Elderly people, especially if they already suffer from processes of cognitive decline, obviously have great difficulties in adapting to changes in, or may have completely lost the ability to, restructure their environment and social relationships. Change of residence in old age as a specific risk factor for depression or confusional states also illustrates the model assumption that certain mental disorders in old age result from a failure of individual coping skills (24).

In the last few years the importance of emotional and cognitive skills in coping with crises, life-altering events, and chronic disease has been established in several studies conducted with various age groups (25–29). A person's coping resources, i.e. his coping strategies and past experience, seem to play a central part in mastering crises and stressful situations without becoming mentally ill. Although, apart from a few exceptions (30, 31), the coping behaviours of elderly people have not yet been sufficiently studied, several factors seem to indicate that the remaining coping resources of the elderly consist of personality factors that mediate, to a considerable extent, the influence of life-altering events that require considerable readjustment and put the elderly at risk for mental disorders.

Social isolation and social support in old age

Several studies (10, 13, 32–34) investigating the close association between insufficient social support and depression and elevated risk for other mental and physical disorders as well seem to indicate that in old age, too, adequate social support, in both quantitative and qualitative terms, favourably influences physical and mental health. Only a few studies, however, have been devoted specifically to this question. Moreover, the existing studies have focused on social isolation rather than social support as an independent variable. Lowenthal and co-workers (35, 36) in San Francisco, Reimann & Häfner (37), in Mannheim, and Dalgard (38), in Oslo, found a high frequency of mental disorder among elderly people living in social isolation. Cooper & Sosna (39), in the previously mentioned study conducted in Mannheim, were able to prove this association only in part: living alone (in one-person households) was not associated with a higher frequency of mental disorders among the Mannheim elderly population. Most elderly people are obviously capable of maintaining an adequate number of social contacts by various means of communication, e.g. the telephone. In addition, Lowenthal and Cooper & Sosna found a small number of elderly people, mainly males, who lived rather isolated lives before and after reaching old age, but who did not seem to suffer from it; so long as they were free from physical disability, they did not seem to depend on social contacts or social support. The frequency of functional mental disorders was found to be clearly higher among elderly people who had considerable deficits in social contacts and social integration and had a subjective feeling of loneliness.

The relationships between the quality and quantity of social networks and health risks in old age are obviously complex and in need of further research.

New aspects of social support research

Although there are more of less comparable research findings indicating that social support either exerts a direct, favourable influence on the maintenance of physical and mental health or buffers against the adverse effects of stressful life events and against depression, the various studies conducted can hardly be compared in view of the differences in their conceptualization of social support.

According to Lin & colleagues (15), social support arises from the relationships a person has with other individuals, groups, or society. Cobb (10) stresses the subjective component, defining social support as the information indicating to a person that he is loved, cared for, and esteemed and that he belongs to a system of mutual obligations and social roles. George (40) differentiates between the interaction patterns within social networks operating in everyday situations and those operating in crises. Thoits (41) differentiates social support according to the amount, quality, type, and source of the support received. According to Pearlin and co-workers (42), social support provides access to other individuals and groups in coping with the vicissitudes of life. Still other investigators make a distinction between objective and subjective components of social support (11, 12) or propose still finer differentiations on the basis of empirical analyses (43–45).

On the basis of the various definitions and usages of the concept of social support in the empirical literature, a number of differentiations can be made (21).

We can distinguish between an objective and an interactional dimension of social support. The objective dimension refers to parameters such as the size and extension of the immediate personal network, the density of and the cohesion within the network, the ratio between relatives and non-relatives within the network, and the direction of the relationships. The interactional dimension concerns the actual utilization of these relationships. It can be broken down according to the type of support, the underlying roles of the various components of the network, and assessment of the support received.

Social support can also be differentiated according to its type – as crisis support, instrumental help, emotional support, or everyday support, in the sense of social interconnectedness and participation in joint activities.

Differentiation of these various dimensions of social support is necessary in order to be better able to compare the existing studies with each other and to analyze the beneficial effects of the various dimensions of the theoretical concept of social support in crisis situations. The interactions within social networks not only further social support but also mediate purely instrumental help or, as social reference groups, contribute to the establishment of behavioural norms and, in some cases, also to the adoption of deviant norms.

Social networks and the lay referral system

Especially in countries and areas with inadequate professional health services, lay referral systems play an important role in the counselling, care, and nursing of the sick. Even in countries with comparatively well developed service structures, according to a study conducted by Fry (46), 75 % of all morbid episodes, rheumatic complaints, respiratory illnesses, mental disorders, and skin diseases, in particular, are treated within the lay referral system. The decision as to when a complaint has grown severe enough to consult a doctor is also made within this system.

In a study carried out in New York, Suchman (47) found that 75 % of the persons interviewed had discussed their symptoms with other people, usually relatives, before consulting medical services. The finding of Both & Babchu (48) (investigating the factors underlying the decision to consult a doctor) that two-thirds of those interviewed regarded the advice of relatives and friends as very crucial in their decision to consult medical services illustrates the importance of personal confidants in help-seeking behaviour for illness. Such studies also indicate that the assessment of illness is based not only on the subjective experience of the persons concerned but also on whether that experience is confirmed and thus rendered objective by the other people contacted.

Social networks as normative reference groups

The influence social networks have on the decision to consult medical services suffices to illustrate their importance as normative reference groups. If early advice to consult a doctor is based on responsible and health-conscious behaviour, such advice cannot be expected in a primary group in which physician-averse attitudes predominate. In such cases, hesitation, unsuccessful lay therapy, and too-late advice to turn to a medical service may have a deteriorating and damaging effect on a person's health.

In the genesis of certain categories of mental disorder, such as crisis reactions or drug abuse, in hysterical symptoms, or in suicidal behaviour, processes of social influence emanating from primary groups frequently play a role. The diffusion of drug abuse among adolescents is unlikely without their membership in a reference group of drug-using peers. It is within this subcultural climate that the deviant behaviour of drug abuse is learned and maintained through mechanisms of mutual strengthening of behaviour and threat of punishment. Even the quality of a pleasant experience in the subjective situation of intoxication is often reached only through processes of learning. In many cases the first experiences with drugs are physically unpleasant and ambiguous. Very frequently the new users would not continue to take drugs if they did not learn to redefine these experiences as pleasant (49). They will be the more prone to do so the less they want to lose the personal contact with the group and the more they have lost contact with the dominant culture.

The importance of membership in a peer group in the initiation to use drugs has been demonstrated in various interviews. Only a few adolescents start to experiment with drugs on their own initiative, whereas 90% to 95% of those interviewed who had had experiences with drugs had had their first contacts in the company of friends, who had introduced them to drug-taking (50–52). The importance of peer groups as normative reference groups has also been emphasized by Andrews & Kandel (53), who have observed a presocialization process in people who start to take drugs, in the sense of their having adopted the attitudes and ways of thinking of those who have already practised the habit for a longer time.

Further well-known examples of the functioning of behavioural models and the effects they may have are short-term occurrences of hysterical symptoms, which in many cases have affected entire classes of pupils, peer groups, or groups of workers in factories (54).

Among people who had attempted suicide, Kreitman, Smith, & Tan (55) found a four times higher incidence rate than expected of earlier suicide attempts in their primary groups. These investigators explain this finding by social influence and the fact that people with suicidal behaviour frequently act as models for others. These findings might be interpreted in another way as well, namely, that people with a predisposition to suicidal behaviour often select each other as friends. The results of a study conducted by Phillips (56, 57), however, clearly support the theory of social influence on suicidal behaviour. Phillips found that in the first four weeks after a front-page story of a suicide, the suicide rate experienced a rise. The rise was the higher the more publicity the case received and the more known the suicide was to the general public. By analogy to the increase after publication of Goethe's essay 'The sorrows of the young Werther', Phillips terms this finding the Werther effect.

Similarly, Welz (58) ascribed the high concentration of attempted suicides in small neighbourhoods in Mannheim to the influence of preceding suicidal attempts by acquaintances and friends: 15% of all suicides attempted by the Mannheim population between 1966 and 1975 concentrated in 71 streets in which only 4.5% of the total Mannheim population lived. For six streets the rate of attempted suicide was over 40/1000 of the population. The 0.4% of the total population living in these six streets accounted for as much as 2.5% of all attempted suicides; and in the street with the highest rate, every 14th inhabitant attempted suicide in the 10-year period from 1966 to 1975.

Summary

Primary groups can further health-conscious behaviour and help considerably in coping with life crises. On the other hand, links with subcultural groups may increase the risk of behavioural disorder.

Although it has received most attention in the psychological literature, the

158   *Heinz Häfner & Rainer Welz*

aid of social networks in coping with crises and protecting against life stress and strainful life events is only one dimension to be taken into account in investigating the relationship between social networks and states of health. There are three dimensions of social risks that have to be considered when examining the importance of social networks for health:

1. their function as a source of social support in coping with crises and life stress;
2. their function as normative reference groups and their influence on behaviour favourable or detrimental to health; and
3. their function as integral parts of lay referrals to medical services.

References

1. Durkheim, E. *Suicide.* New York, The Free Press, 1981.
2. Faris, R. L., & Dunham, W. H. *Mental disorders in urban areas.* Chicago, University of Chicago Press, 1939.
3. Häfner, H., Reimann, H., Immich, H., & Martini, H. Inzidenz seelischer Erkrankungen in Mannheim, 1965. *Social Psychiatry,* 4, 126–35 (1969).
4. Sainsbury, P. *Suicide in London.* London, Chapman & Hall, 1955.
5. Bott, E. *Family and social network. Roles, norms and external relationships in ordinary urban families.* London, Tavistock, 1957.
6. Hammer, M. Social support, social networks and schizophrenia. *Schizophrenia Bulletin,* 7, 45–57 (1981).
7. Pattison, E. M., de Francisco, D., & Wood, P. A psychosocial kinship model for family therapy. *American Journal of Psychiatry,* 132, 1246–48 (1975).
8. Tolsdorf, C. C. Social networks, support and coping. An explanatory study. *Family Process,* 15, 407 (1976).
9. Nuckolls, K. B., Cassel, J. C., & Kaplan, B. Psychosocial assets, life crisis and the prognosis of pregnancy. *American Journal of Epidemiology,* 95, 431–41 (1972).
10. Cobb, S. Social support as a moderator of life stress. *Psychosomatic Medicine,* 38, 300–314 (1976).
11. Andrews, G., Tennant, C., Hewson, D., & Vaillant, G. Life event stress, social support, coping style and risk of psychological impairment. *Journal of Nervous and Mental Disease,* 166, 307–16 (1978).
12. Henderson, A. S., Duncan-Jones, P., Byrne, D. G., & Scott, R. Measuring social relationships. The interviewer schedule for social interaction. *Psychological Medicine,* 10, 723–34 (1980).
13. Brown, G. W., & Harris, T. *Social origins of depression.* London, Tavistock, 1978.
14. Hautzinger, M. Kritische Lebensereignisse, soziale Unterstützung und Depressivität bei älteren Menschen. *Zeitschrift Für Klinische Psychologie und Psychotherapie,* 1, 1–11 (1985).
15. Lin, N., Simeone, R., Ensel, W., & Kuo, W. Social support, stressful life events

and illness. A model and an empirical test. *Journal of Health and Social Behavior,* **20**, 108–19 (1979).

16. Miller, P. M., & Ingham, J. G. Friends, confidants and symptoms. *Social Psychiatry,* **11**, 51–58 (1976).

17. Siegrist, J., Dittmann, K., Rittner, K., & Weber, J. *Soziale Belastungen und Herzinfarkt. Eine medizinsoziologische Fall-Kontroll-Studie.* Stuttgart, Enke, 1980.

18. Häfner, H. Mental health in the elderly. *Interdisciplinary Science Review,* **11**(2), 202–210 (1986).

19. Clayton, P. J. Mortality and morbidity in the first years of widowhood. *Archives of General Psychiatry,* **30**, 747–50 (1974).

20. Clayton, P. J. The sequelae and nonsequelae of conjugal bereavement. *American Journal of Psychiatry,* **136**, 1530–34 (1976).

21. Veiel, H. O. F. Dimensions of social support: A conceptual framework. *Social Psychiatry,* **20**, 156–62 (1985).

22. Diekstra, R. F. W. Psychological and social aspects of mental health in the elderly: A summarizing co-lecture. In H. Häfner, G. Moschel, & N. Sartorius (Eds.), *Mental health in the elderly. A review of the present state of research.* Berlin, Springer, 1986.

23. Häfner, H. *Psychische Gesundheit im Alter.* Stuttgard, Gustav Fischer Verlag, 1986.

24. Kanowski, S. Community care for psychiatric patients. In H. Häfner, G. Moschel, & N. Sartorius (Eds.), *Mental health in the elderly. A review of the present state of research.* Berlin, Springer, 1986.

25. Liebermann, M. Adaption processes in late life. In N. Datan, & H. Ginsberg (Eds.), *Normative life crisis.* New York, Academic Press, 1975.

26. Verwoerdt, A. *Clinical gerontopsychiatry.* Baltimore, Williams & Wilkins, 1976.

27. Wheaton, B. Stress, personal coping resources, and psychiatric symptoms: An investigation of interactive models. *Journal of Health and Social Behavior,* **24**, 208–229 (1983).

28. Menaghan, E. G. Individual coping efforts: Moderators of the relationship between life stress and mental health outcomes. In H. B. Kaplan (Ed.), *Psychosocial stress.* New York, Academic Press, 1983. Pp. 159–91.

29. Pearlin, L. J., & Schooler, C. The structure of coping. *Journal of Health and Social Behaviour,* **19**, 2–21 (1978).

30. Lazarus, R. S., & Olbrich, E. Problems of stress and coping in old age. In M. Bergener *et al.* (Eds.), *Problems of stress and coping in old age.* New York, Springer, 1983. Pp. 272–87.

31. Lazarus, R. S., & Delongis, A. Psychological stress and coping in aging. *American Psychologist,* **38**, 245–54 (1983).

32. Dohrenwend, B. S. (Ed.) *Stressful life events and their context.* New York, Neale Watson Academic Publications, 1981.

33. Surtees, P. J. Social support, residual adversity and depressive outcome. *Social Psychiatry,* **15**, 71–80 (1980).

34. Surtees, P. J., & Ingham, J. G. Life stress and social outcome: Application of a dissipation model to life events. *Social Psychiatry,* **15**, 21–31 (1980).

160   *Heinz Häfner & Rainer Welz*

35. Lowenthal, M. F. The relationship between social factors and mental health in the aged. In A. Simon & L. J. Epstein (Eds.), *Aging in modern society*. Psychiatric Research Reports of the American Psychiatric Association, No. 23. Washington, DC, American Psychiatric Association, 1968. Pp. 161–69.
36. Lowenthal, M. F., & Berkman, P. L. *Aging and mental disorders in San Francisco*. San Francisco, Jossey-Bass, 1967.
37. Reimann, H., & Häfner, H. Psychische Erkrankungen alter Menschen in Mannheim. Eine Untersuchung zur Konsultationsinzidenz. *Social Psychiatry, 7*, 53–69 (1972).
38. Dalgard, O. S. Mental health, neighbourhood and related social variables in Oslo. *Acta Psychiatrica Scandinavica, 285*, 298–304 (1980).
39. Cooper, B., & Sosna, U. Psychische Erkrankungen in der Altenbevölkerung. Eine epidemiologische Feldstudie in Mannheim. *Nervenarzt, 54*, 239–49 (1983).
40. George, K. K. *Role transitions in later life*. Monterrey, CA, Brooks/Cole, 1980.
41. Thoits, P. A. Conceptual, methodological and theoretical problems in studying social support as a buffer against stress. *Journal of Health and Social Behavior, 23*, 145–59 (1982).
42. Pearlin, L. J., Lieberman, M., Menaghan, E., & Mullan, J. The stress process. *Journal of Health and Social Behavior, 22*, 337–56 (1981).
43. Norbeck, J. S., & Tilden, V. P. Life stress, social support and emotional disequilibrium in complication of pregnancy: A prospective multivariate study. *Journal of Health and Social Behavior, 24*, 30–46 (1983).
44. Schaefer, C., Coyne, J. C., & Lazarus, R. S. The health related functions of social support. *Journal of Behavioral Medicine, 4*, 381–406 (1981).
45. Monroe, S. M., Innhoff, D. F., Wise, B. D., & Harris, J. E. Predictions of psychological symptoms under high risk psychosocial circumstances: Life events, social support and symptom specificity. *Journal of Abnormal Psychology, 92*, 338–50 (1983).
46. Fry, J. *A new approach to medicine. Priorities and principles of health care*. Baltimore, University Park Press, 1978.
47. Suchman, E. Social patterns and medical care. *Journal of Health and Human Behavior, 6*, 2–16 (1965).
48. Booth, A., & Babchuk, N. Seeking health care from new resources. *Journal of Health and Social Behavior, 13*, 90–99 (1972).
49. Becker, H. S. *Outsiders. Studies in the sociology of deviance*. New York, Academic Press, 1966.
50. Kandel, D. Interpersonal influence on adolescent illegal drug use. In E. Josephson & E. Carroll (Eds.), *Drug use: Epidemiological and sociological approaches*. Washington, DC, Hemisphere, 1974. Pp. 207–240.
51. Tec, N. The peergroup and marihuana use. *Crime and Delinquency, 18*, 298–309 (1972).
52. Zimmermann, R. Zur Situation des ersten Rauschmittelkonsums. In K. H. Reuband (Ed.), *Rauschmittelkonsum. Soziale Abweichung und institutionelle Reaktion*. Wiesbaden, Westd Verlag, 1976. Pp. 63–76.

53. Andrews, K. H., & Kandel, D. B. Attitude and behavior: A specification of the contingent consistency theory. *American Sociological Review*, **44**, 298–310 (1979).

54. Kerckhoff, A. C., & Back, K. W. *The June bug: A study of hysterical contagion.* New York, Appleton-Century-Crofts, 1968.

55. Kreitman, N., Smith, P., & Tan, E. Atempted suicide as language: An empirical study. *British Journal of Psychiatry*, **116**, 465–73 (1970).

56. Phillips, B. P. The influence of suggestion on suicide: Substantive and theoretical implications of the Werther effect. *American Sociological Review*, **39**, 340–54 (1974).

57. Phillips, B. P. Motor vehicle fatalities increase just after publicized suicide stories. *Science*, **196**, 1464–65 (1977).

58. Welz, R. *Selbstmordversuche in städtischen Lebensumwelten.* Weinheim, Beltz, 1979.

59. Welz, R., Veiel, H. & Häfner, H. Social Support and Suicidal Behaviour. In H. Möller, A. Schmidtke & R. Welz (Eds.) *Current Issues of Suicidology*, Heidelberg, New York, Springer (1988).

7

Mental health aspects of general health care

David Goldberg

In recent years the advent of standardized psychiatric research interviews and operational criteria for psychiatric diagnoses has been accompanied by a flurry of scientific papers reporting the prevalence of mental disorders among patients receiving care from general practitioners, internists, and surgeons. It has become clear that mental disorders are not only very much more common in health care settings than in random samples of the population but also that they are frequently unrecognized by medical professionals.

Prevalence and recognition of mental disorders among medical and surgical inpatients

The past 25 years have seen the appearance of numerous surveys of the mental health of patients in the medical and surgical wards of general hospitals. Lipowski (1) reviewed ten studies and found that the average number of such patients with a mental disorder constituted 49% (SD, 23.1). Since the time of his study (1967), operational definitions of mental illness have become available for research use, and these have resulted in somewhat lower figures. Nevertheless, most recent surveys confirm that between one-fourth and one-third of patients on medical and surgical wards have diagnosable mental illnesses and that a substantial proportion of such illnesses are not detected by medical staff.

Schwab and co-workers (2), using the Beck Depression Inventory and the Hamilton Rating Scale for depression on a sample of 153 patients on various medical wards in Florida, found that between 22% and 23% of the patients were depressed. These investigators observed that the medical staff diagnosed depression four times more frequently among upper-class patients than among the others although the condition was equally common in all classes. Moreover, depression was diagnosed among both the severely and the mildly physically ill and in all age groups. It was almost as frequent among men as among women,

The author is Professor of Psychiatry, University of Manchester, Manchester, England.

though in women it was expressed somatically whereas men displayed despair. These depressive illnesses were often missed by the medical staff because of the pressure of other work, or because 'zeal in pursuing interesting diseases during the work-up seemed to block the physician's sensitivity to emotional components'.

The same measures were used by Moffic & Paykel (3) in a study of 150 medical inpatients in New Haven, Connecticut. These investigators found that clinically significant depression was present in 24% of the patients within a week of admission and developed in a further 5% during their hospital stay. The medical clinicians observed no mental abnormality whatever in 53% of these depressed patients, noted the depression in only 14%, and offered treatment to only 9%. Moffic & Paykel comment that the aetiology of the depression tended to be closely related to the physical illness for which the patients were receiving care. Depression was more common in the severely ill and in those who had been ill for some time or whose alertness was diminished. When compared with nondepressed patients, those with depression were less likely to be discharged home and were more likely to die. The largest group (65%) were those in whom the depression appeared to be a consequence of the physical illness; in a further 21% the depression had clearly antedated the physical illness: life stress appeared to have been followed by depression, and then by somatic illness. The rest of the patients had a depressive illness that caused physical symptoms rather than actual disease.

Maguire and associates (4) used a screening questionnaire (the GHQ-60), followed by a standardized psychiatric assessment, with 230 medical inpatients in Oxford, England. They found that 23% of the patients were mentally ill, 80% of the diagnoses being affective illnesses; a further 13%, organic psychosyndromes; and the remainder, alcoholism or personality disorders. The medical staff recognized the existence of these problems in fewer than half the patients (49%), and had failed to refer many patients who might have benefited from psychiatric treatment. Patients tended to be referred if they were weepy and agitated, complained excessively, were very noisy, or refused to cooperate in treatment. When Hawton (5) followed these patients up 18 months later, those who had been mentally unwell at the time of the original survey had a higher mortality rate or tended to have persistent mental problems over the period of follow-up.

Bridges & Goldberg (6) used the GHQ-28 and the Clinical Interview Schedule with 100 neurological inpatients in Manchester, England, and found diagnosable mental illnesses in 27% of the male patients and 53% of the females. The neurologists, however, identified mental disorders in only 10% of the men and 11% of the women. The patients were interviewed just before their discharge from the hospital and were asked whether the neurologists had enquired about their mood. It was found that such enquiries were more frequent for male patients, and this was believed to account for the low detection rate for female patients.

It was disturbing to find that the neurologists were no more likely to have asked about mood in those with a mental illness than in those without one, which suggests that the clinicians were not alert to the cues indicative of emotional illness. The research psychiatrist asked all patients in this study whether they would have minded an enquiry about mood from the neurologists; about 58% of the mentally ill and exactly half of the others wished that such an enquiry had been made. It was of interest that a substantial minority of those with mental illnesses would not have liked to discuss their problems on the open ward and colluded with their doctors by regarding the purpose of their hospital stay as alleviation of the physical causes of their symptoms. These same patients, however, readily discussed their mental symptoms with the psychiatrist in the privacy of the interview room.

Patients with specific disorders

A number of studies have dealt with patients with specific disorders. For example, Fras and co-workers (7) found depression in 76% of patients with carcinoma of the pancreas – a much higher rate than was discovered for other abdominal neoplasms. Lobo & associates[1] screened 110 patients in a cancer centre with the GHQ-30 and the Present State Examination and found 57% to have mental illnesses, of which only 44% were recognized by the clinicians. Rabins & Brooks (8) used the GHQ-28, followed by the Present State Examination, with a population of 25 patients with multiple sclerosis and found over half of them had a mental disorder. Lloyd & Cawley (9), using the Clinical Interview Schedule, assessed 100 consecutive men one week after their first myocardial infarction and determined that 35% were suffering from a mental illness, which in 46% of them had antedated the heart attack.

Case finding by screening test

All the above studies have relied on assessment by a research clinician using a standardized interview as the case-finding procedure. Many other investigators have merely administered screening tests to medical or surgical patients without going to the additional trouble and expense of direct clinical assessment. It is, of course, foolish to equate a high score on a screening test with the presence of a disorder, not only because of the presence of false positives and false negatives but because the threshold score used to discriminate between potentially normal subjects and potential cases of mental illness needs to be adjusted to take account of each of the consulting settings. This is true of any screening test. Nevertheless, such studies have confirmed the findings already reported for neurological patients (10) and those on haemodialysis (11) and have suggested high rates for dermatological inpatients (12) and those with rheumatoid arthritis (13) or with severe burns (14).

Prevalence of mental disorders among ambulatory medical patients
In 1960 Culpan & Davies (*15*), using unstandardized clinical assessments, reviewed 11 studies of mental illness among medical outpatients and reported an average prevalence of 27.3% (SD, 13.2). More recent surveys have used research interviews and have broadly confirmed these early findings. Four studies have used the Clinical Interview Schedule (CIS) and found a prevalence of 34% among medical outpatients (*16*), 20% among patients attending a venereal disease clinic (*17*), 44% among patients at a cardiac clinic in Spain (*18*), and 31% among patients on home haemodialysis (*19*). A further study used the Present State Examination to reveal a prevalence of emotional illness of 29% among gynaecological outpatients (*20*). Numerous studies have employed psychiatric screening tests supplemented by second-stage case-finding interviews to estimate prevalence (*21, 22*), but such studies should be regarded with caution, for reasons already mentioned.

Similar findings are reported for primary care settings. Goldberg & Blackwell (*23*), using the Clinical Interview Schedule, reported that 30% of consecutive patients seen in a South London general practice were mentally ill; and Skuse & Williams (*24*), with the same instrument, have recently reported a figure of 34% for a practice in the same area. In the United States, Goldberg and co-workers (*25*), also using the Clinical Interview Schedule, found a prevalence of mental disorder of 35% in five practices in Philadelphia, Pennsylvania. And Hoeper and associates (*26*), using the 'SADS-L' interview (*27*), found a prevalence of 27% in Marshfield, Wisconsin.

Recognition of mental illness among medical outpatients
There is abundant evidence that minor mental illness is not well recognized by medical practitioners. In a study by Brody (*21*), 58 participating doctors diagnosed such illnesses in 41.7% of 235 medical outpatients, yet one can calculate a probable prevalence of 71.8% (*28, 29*), indicating that only 58% of the illnesses were recognized. This figure is close to the 55% recognition of mental illnesses found by Marks & co-workers (*30*) in a survey of 91 family physicians in Manchester, England. Nielsen & Williams (*31*) reported that physicians failed to diagnose 57% of depressive illnesses occurring in 526 medical outpatients in Washington State, USA. Chancellor and associates (*32*) found that Australian family doctors failed to detect 73% of patients who, as judged by a psychiatric screening questionnaire, probably had a mental illness.

Patients who have mental illnesses that are not detected by their doctors have been termed the 'hidden psychiatric morbidity' of general medical practice. They fall into two main groups. First are the patients whose mental illness accompanies a physical disease; the former may be secondary to the latter, or be unrelated to it. In either case, the presence of the physical illness serves to draw the physician's attention and care away from the patient's mental condition. The second group is made up of patients whose mental illnesses are presented as physical symptoms – 'somatic presentations' of mental illness. Approximately half of the mental illnesses seen in community settings are accompanied by significant somatic symptoms (33), and these symptoms also tend to 'distract' the physician and focus his attention and treatment on those symptoms.

Many physicians attempt to make single diagnoses of their patients, and this causes them to make two potentially serious errors: they tend to ignore a mental disorder once a physical diagnosis has been made, and they wrongly assume that the patients for whom they have been unable to make a physical diagnosis are probably mentally/emotionally ill. It is of interest that in Bridges & Goldberg's study of neurological patients (6), those for whom the neurologists could not make a confident diagnosis were no more likely to be mentally ill than those with undoubted neurological disorders.

Relationships between mental disorders and physical symptoms

Recent community surveys have indicated that somewhere between 9% and 12% of the population can be expected to be mentally ill at a particular time (33). Since mentally disordered people can become physically ill for the same reasons as mentally healthy people, we should expect to find some patients in general medical settings with two unrelated illnesses, and this certainly does happen. A study under way in my own unit shows that the mental illnesses in such cases are particularly unlikely to be detected by the medical staff, for understandable reasons. Yet every survey mentioned above reports rates of mental disorder greatly in excess of what might have been expected by chance. That mentally disordered people are generally likely to select themselves for medical care seems not to be the explanation, as Cooper and colleagues' (34) survey of women undergoing elective sterilization indicates: their rate of mental morbidity was exactly the same as that of a group of randomly selected women, both before surgery and 18 months later.

There are, in fact, five kinds of relationship between mental and physical symptoms that account for the high rate of association between the two.

First, a mental disorder may provoke or release physical disease. It is a clinical commonplace that painful conditions such as migraine may be released by a depressive illness; and in many of the surveys already cited (3, 4, 9), the mental disorder preceded the onset of physical disease in some of the patients. The evidence concerning psychological antecedents of physical disease is inconclusive, but several studies have suggested lines that are worth pursuing. Schmale & Iker (35) showed that the depressive symptom of hopelessness predicted cervical cancer in women undergoing routine cervical smear examinations. Murphy & Brown (36) found that when episodes of organic illness were preceded by traumatic life events, the connecting link was likely to be a mild affective illness. This seems to fit in with Craig's (37) finding that frustrating life events may be followed by symptoms of tension and irritability, and then by the onset of organic disease. There is also some evidence that depression may put men at greater risk of developing cancer (*38*), but some other studies have not confirmed this (*39*).

Second, the mental symptoms may be the presenting symptoms of a physical disease. Muhangi (*40*) describes how typhoid fever may present as a mental disorder in Uganda; and there are, of course, many diseases – such as myxoedema and pernicious anaemia – that can present with mental symptoms. However, such cases, although theoretically interesting, are rare.

Third, the mental illness may be a direct consequence of physical disease, as in the depressive illnesses that follow the diagnosis of cancer (*41*, *42*), which may be related to chronic pain, to the patient's sense of hopelessness, or to severe physical disability. In such patients the presence of undoubted physical disease seems to dominate the physician's attention and to distract him from the mental distress.

Fourth, mental illness may exacerbate the pain of a physical disease. Patients who are depressed experience pain and discomfort more intensely even when they are well. This is true of any chronic pain, from sciatica to that associated with malignant disease. In ambulant settings patients may seek help for minor symptoms, such as tinnitus, that they appear to tolerate easily when they are well.

Finally, mental illness may present to doctors with physical symptoms that have no organic basis. This is the phenomenon of 'somatization' of psychic distress, and it is easily the most important reason for the excess rates of mental illness found among medical patients. There are two studies that indicate that in such patients it is possible that the mental disorder forms a connecting link between stressful life events – usually ones involving loss – and physical ill health. Creed (*43*) found that patients with a normal appendix removed because of abdominal pain were twice as likely to be mentally ill as either patients with inflamed appendices or normal subjects, and very much more likely to have experienced a severe or threatening life event in the 13 weeks preceding the operation. Craig (*37*) has extended these observations and shown that traumatic life events are often followed by typical affective illnesses that present with somatic symptoms without organic pathology.

Somatic presentations of mental disorder

Somatization has been succinctly defined as the expression of personal and social distress in an idiom of bodily complaints for which medical help is sought (*44*). This is a fairly broad definition since it includes somatic symptoms unaccompanied by affective symptoms. In the research carried out in my own unit, *somatization* refers to patients who present to doctors with somatic symptoms, but who report other symptoms that permit psychiatric diagnoses to be made on the basis of research criteria. In practice, these patients are depressed, anxious, or both. Katon & co-workers (*45*) apply a broader definition and include 'the use of somatic symptoms in the absence of physical disease *to avoid dysphoric affect*' and 'psychophysiological

symptoms secondary to stressful life events with minimization of the life problems
that have precipitated the illness'. It is clear that neither of the latter groups of
patients would have diagnosable mental illnesses. Whichever definition is used, it
is essential to grasp that the concept is very much wider than the 'Somatoform
Disorders' in the third edition of the American Psychiatric Association's *Diagnostic
and statistical manual of mental disorders* (DSM-III); indeed, the DSM-III disorders
accounted for only 21% of the 'somatizers' in Katon and colleagues' study.

Somatization is a worldwide phenomenon, even more common in developing
than in industrialized countries. Marsella (46) has shown that somatic presentations
of depression are more frequent in non-Western than in Western culture. High
rates have been reported for Saudi Arabia (47), Iraq (48), West Africa (49, 50),
India (51), Taiwan (52), Hong Kong (53), Peru (54), and Uganda (55). It should
not be thought, however, that somatization is uncommon in the West. In terms
of prevalence, somatic symptoms were present in 50% of the mental disorders
detected in primary care settings in London (56) and in 52% of those seen in
Philadelphia (33). If the analysis is confined to patients presenting with new episodes of illness, 60% of those seen in primary care in Manchester in which a
DSM-III diagnosis of mental illness can be made will be found to be presented
somatically (57).

Somatization is clearly an important phenomenon, so it is reasonable to ask
why it has taken so long to discover it. One of the reasons must be that in many
countries, mental patients are segregated, and this often means that psychiatrists
are segregated as well. Their clinical practice consists of patients referred to them
by their colleagues or who choose to come themselves. Patients whose mental
illness is expressed somatically are neither referred by psychiatrists' medical
colleagues nor seek psychiatric care themselves. Their doctors all too often see
their task as eliminating physical pathology, and the patients typically consider
themselves physically ill. Another reason must be that such patients cannot easily
be fitted into the existing taxonomies of neurosis. However, now that consultation
liaison services are being developed in the West, and mental health services in the
rest of the world, psychiatry is belatedly acknowledging a phenomenon that is
considerably older than the overtly psychological presentations that have become
more common in the West.

When Beard (58), in 1880, originally described neurasthenia, he regarded it
as a specifically American disorder. Though DSM-III has now 'abolished' this
disorder, its symptoms continue to be very common – in the United States and
elsewhere. Patients whom Beard would have called neurasthenics, and who are
still thus described in the People's Republic of China and in the Soviet Union,
are, according to DSM-III, suffering from 'major depressive disorder'. Kleinman
(59), using Spitzer's 'SADS' interview (27), studied 100 patients with 'neurasthenia' seen in Hunan, China, and allowed more than one diagnosis per patient.

Depression was diagnosed in 93% (major depressive disorder, in 87%), anxiety-related disorders, in 69%; somatoform disorders, in only 25%; culture-bound syndromes, in only 14%; and chronic pain syndromes, in 44%. The ubiquity of depressive symptoms diagnosable by DSM-III criteria does not mean that the patients were 'really' depressed. They *really* had neurasthenic symptoms, and these symptoms were broadly similar to those described by Beard a century ago.

Kleinman & Kleinman (44) argue, correctly, that 'neurasthenia' and 'depression' are the distinctive ways in which the same psychobiological state is construed by current Chinese and American cultures in both lay and professional concepts of distress. In China, the concept 'neurasthenia' emphasizes the supposed biological basis of the disorder and reduces the stigma that attaches to mental illness in that country (all the patients *had* experienced dysphoric emotions, but they suppressed them and, in consulting health professionals, emphasized physical symptoms).

The disadvantages of the label 'neurasthenic' are that it distracts attention from the social, psychological, and communicative aspects of the disorder, and certainly leads to frequent consultations and polypharmacy (the patients were receiving, on average, five different drugs). The Western concept 'depressive illness' gives primacy to the mood component of the syndrome and leads to prescription of mood-enhancing medication. However, the possibility that antidepressant drugs may affect symptoms other than mood tends to be ignored, and symptoms that cannot plausibly be related to the patient's mood tend to be neglected. Katon & co-workers (60) have pointed out that even when patients whose illness is expressed somatically have had their mood enhanced by antidepressants, their patterns of abnormal behaviour may have become stabilized by the secondary gains of the symptoms and the way in which their illness has been treated. Somatization is often encouraged and rewarded by physicians.

Katon & colleagues (60) have argued that somatization is associated in the West with lower socioeconomic and educational levels, rural origins, and active religious affiliation. Nemiah & Sifneos (61) have advanced the hypothesis that patients who express emotional problems in somatic terms may lack a vocabulary of emotion − a condition they term *alexithymia*. Although such patients may be represented in Katon's group of 'somatizers' without overt affective disturbance, it is important to emphasize that the vast majority of such patients have a copious vocabulary of emotion: they just use the language of pains and other somatic symptoms as well. Typically, they are concerned mainly with their somatic symptoms, and they often do not connect their mental/emotional symptoms with their principal complaints.

I follow Rosen (62) in categorizing somatization according to its course:

Acute somatization consists of psychophysiological symptoms brought on by autonomic overarousal in response to life stress. Somatization occurs when the patient, often abetted by his family, systematically focuses on psychophysiological symptoms rather than any affective or cognitive components. Treatment should consist of reassurance and explanation, with occasional use of short-term anxiolytics.

In *subacute somatization*, the somatic symptoms are most often part of an affective illness, with symptoms of anxiety, depression, and neurasthenia. The first step in the management of patients with this condition is to encourage them to construe their complaints differently so that they can see the connection between the mental and the physical; the second is to learn what has happened in their lives to produce their symptoms. Most of these patients meet DSM-III criteria for major depressive disorder, and it is reasonable to prescribe antidepressant medication — usually a sedating preparation. The physician should, at follow-up visits, try to discuss the social and interpersonal setting in which the disorder is occurring.

In *chronic somatization* there are established affective symptoms, so the patients meet the criteria for major depressive disorder, generalized anxiety disorder, dysthymic disorder, or even one of the somatoform disorders. Since the symptoms are part of the patients' way of relating to other people and of their coping style, treatment by a psychotropic drug alone usually will not suffice to eliminate the symptoms or reduce the behaviour that has caused the patients to seek care. The abnormal behaviour associated with the illness may have been rewarded by medical personnel and by the patient's family, and intervention should be aimed at helping the patient readjust to the demands of his or her environment.

The management of mental illness in medical settings
There is enormous variation among individual physicians both in their ability to detect mental illness and in the kind of treatment they give patients with particular disorders. The overall picture affords no grounds for complacency. Benzodiazepines are commonly prescribed in medical settings, yet major depressive disorder is the most common single diagnosis. In many parts of the world, no liaison psychiatric service is available; and even when psychiatrists *are* available, they often are not called in to see patients. Steinberg and co-workers (63), in the United States, examined 50 cases of mental illness that had been detected by junior medical staff but that the consultant physician intended to manage without psychiatric help. The investigators asked the physician why he did not intend to seek such help. The reason most often was that the patient 'wasn't crazy'; the next, that the patient would be upset if referred; and the third, that psychiatry could not help. In this study the psychiatrist obtained permission to see these patients despite the lack of a request to that effect and was able to help 80% of those he saw.

Mezey & Kellett (64) conducted a comparable study in England and found that the most common reason why surgeons and physicians in British general hospitals did not refer their patients to psychiatrists was the notion that the patient would dislike such a referral; the next, the stigma attached to being thought mentally ill;

and the third, the inadequacy of local facilities. In some of the hospitals surveyed, the relationship between the psychiatrists and their colleagues was poor; nevertheless, fewer than 20% said they did not refer cases of mental illness because 'any doctor should be able to treat such illnesses'.

It should not be assumed that the situation is any better in primary care settings. Shepherd and his colleagues (65) have written: 'Treatment of minor psychiatric disorders in general practice is often haphazard and inadequate. This state of affairs seemed in many cases to be as unsatisfactory to the doctors concerned as to their patients.' There was a gap between theory and practice. When the general practitioners in the survey were asked how they would treat a series of patients described in brief vignettes, psychotherapy by the general practitioner himself was frequently chosen as the correct management. But when the records of their identified 'psychiatric' patients were examined, the three most common treatments were: 'No treatment recorded', sedatives, and reassurance. The type of treatment offered was related to the age and sex of the patients. For instance, women were more likely to be given sedatives, tranquillizers, or antidepressants, whereas men were apt to receive nothing. The use of tablets of all sorts increased with increasing age of the patients; and advice, reassurance, psychotherapy by the general practitioner, or psychiatric referral became less likely with increasing age.

Johnson (66) interviewed 73 patients who had recently seen their family doctors because of a new episode of mental illness and compared information derived from the doctors' records with that obtained from the patients themselves by psychiatric interview at home. Only two patients had specifically been offered psychotherapy, and neither of these returned to see his doctor. Despite the fact that the patients generally held their doctors in high regard, only 15% of them acknowledged any personal help or support in their illness, and a further 12% thought that their doctors' attitudes had been unhelpful. Though stress factors were highly correlated with the observed outcome in the patients' clinical condition, no doctor had attempted to modify the precipitating factors in any way, and no social agencies had been involved in the treatment of any of the patients. The situation was little better insofar as antidepressant medication was concerned: only 72% had had antidepressants prescribed in what are usually regarded as therapeutic doses, and of these, 59% had ceased taking their medication within 21 days – almost always without the doctor's knowledge.

In a further study with a larger sample, Johnson (67) concluded that even among good family doctors in the Manchester area, knowledge of and interest in psychiatry were strictly limited, and that psychotropic drugs were often inappropriately prescribed, or prescribed in inadequate doses. Another worrying feature was the high proportion of patients on medication for more than three months who were given repeated prescriptions without seeing their doctor.

In a study carried out for the Medical Research Council, Rawnsley, Loudon, & Miles (*68*) came to broadly similar conclusions in a survey of a sample of Welsh country doctors:

> The majority say that they find their psychiatric work irksome by comparison with other aspects of practice, mainly because of the considerable time demanded by psychiatric problems and because of the uncertain and comparatively poor response to their efforts. They are, in the main, apprehensive of any potential increase in the number of chronic psychiatric cases under their care in the community. Drugs form the mainstay of therapy, together with advice and reassurance. Exploratory psychotherapy is rare as a method of treatment; this is not only due to lack of time, but also to serious doubts on the part of the doctors as to the value of such treatment in their hands.

In an Australian study, Brodaty,[2] a trained psychiatrist, sat in with 13 different family doctors and directly observed the treatment given to 239 patients. He comments that their usual strategy was to exclude organic illness, reassure patients, and then treat them symptomatically, often using psychotropic medications inappropriately or inadequately.

Holmes & Speight (*50*) report on the treatment of patients without organic illness among 170 general medical patients in Tanzania's main teaching hospital. Many of these patients appeared emotionally and socially crippled by their illnesses, and some came to dispensaries daily for a long period of time. 'There they receive symptomatic treatment or tranquillisers, but few are cured since their underlying problems, whether social or psychiatric, are not dealt with.' The authors were able to manage these disorders without referral to psychiatrists:

> Some responded well to vigorous reassurance and a physiological explanation of their symptoms, while others required simple psychotherapy. The ability to manage patients successfully in these ways is easily taught, and a diffusion of these skills to all medical and paramedical workers in developing countries is required.

The World Health Organization (*69*) has made great progress in promoting this objective in developing countries (*70*). Murthy (*71*) has reviewed ten training manuals for primary care workers and has produced one that is specifically aimed at mental health problems (*72*). Most of these manuals depend on simple decision trees that lead directly from types of presentation of symptoms to kinds of intervention. Complex examples of such algorithms are provided by Essex & Gosling (*73*), though the examples they give focus on entirely psychological presentations such as violent behaviour, abnormal behaviours, and mood disorders.

Do the mental disorders presented in medical settings matter?

Mental disorders are common in general medical settings, where they usually present with somatic symptoms. When recognized, they are often poorly treated; and when unrecognized, the process of endless physical investigations and symptomatic treatment is likely to reinforce patterns of abnormal behaviour. Johnstone & Goldberg (74) have demonstrated that the provision of psychotherapy and drug treatment for patients with unrecognized mental disorders can shorten the duration of those disorders. An attempt by Hoeper & co-workers (75) to duplicate this finding came to nought, but they were unable to show that the primary care physicians in their study had altered their diagnostic or therapeutic practices as a result of feedback of unexpectedly high scores on a psychiatric screening questionnaire.

Although a number of studies (3, 5, 38, 76) have reported increased mortality among depressed patients with physical illnesses, it is not clear whether terminal disease causes the depression, or vice versa. Querido (77) showed that poor psychosocial adjustment predicted a poor prognosis for patients on the general wards of a hospital, and Cay & co-workers (78) report that a mood disturbance hinders recovery.

Patients whose mental disorders are presented somatically are frequent users of medical services and form a substantial proportion of all patients seen in developing countries. There is evidence that provision of psychiatric care reduces subsequent use of medical services (79–81), so there would appear to be economic as well as humanitarian reasons for improving the detection and treatment of mental disorders in medical settings.

Notes

1. A. Lobo, M. Folstein, & M. Abeloff, Prevalence and recognition of psychiatric morbidity in a cancer center. Unpublished manuscript, Johns Hopkins Hospital, Baltimore, MD, 1979. (Ms available from Dr Folstein.)
2. H. Brodaty, Brief psychotherapy in general practice: A controlled prospective intervention trial. Unpublished MD dissertation, University of New South Wales, Sydney, New South Wales, Australia, 1983.

References

1. Lipowski, Z. J. Review of consultation psychiatry and psychosomatic medicine – 2. *Psychosomatic Medicine*, **29**, 201–224 (1967).
2. Schwab, J., Bialow, M., Brown, J. & Holzer, C. Diagnosing depression in medical inpatients. *Annals of Internal Medicine*, **67**, 695–707 (1967).
3. Moffic, H. & Paykel, E. Depression in medical inpatients. *British Journal of Psychiatry*, **126**, 346–53 (1975).

4. Maguire, P., Julier, D., Hawton, K. & Bancroft, J. Psychiatric morbidity and referral on two medical wards. *British Medical Journal*, **1**, 268–71 (1974).

5. Hawton, K. The long term outcome of psychiatric morbidity detected in general medical patients. *Journal of Psychosomatic Research*, **25**, 237–43 (1981).

6. Bridges, K. & Goldberg, D. Psychiatric illness in neurological inpatients: Patients' views on discussion of emotional problems with neurologists. *British Medical Journal*, **289**, 656–58 (1984).

7. Fras, I., Litin, E. & Pearson, J. Comparison of psychiatric symptoms in carcinoma of the pancreas with those of other intraabdominal neoplasms. *American Journal of Psychiatry*, **123**, 1553–62 (1967).

8. Rabins, P. & Brooks, B. Emotional disturbance in multiple sclerosis patients. *Psychological Medicine*, **11**, 425–27 (1981).

9. Lloyd, G., & Cawley, R. Psychiatric morbidity in men one week after first myocardial infarction. *British Medical Journal*, **2**, 1453–54 (1978).

10. de Paulo, J., Folstein, M. & Gordon, B. Psychiatric screening on a neurological ward. *Psychosomatic Medicine*, **10**, 125–32 (1980).

11. Livesley, W. Psychiatric disturbance and chronic haemodialysis. *British Medical Journal*, **2**, 306 (1979).

12. Hughes, J., Barraclough, B., Hamblin, L. & White, J. Psychiatric symptoms in dermatology patients. *British Journal of Psychiatry*, **143**, 51–54 (1983).

13. Gardiner, B. Psychological aspects of rheumatoid arthritis. *Psychological Medicine*, **10**, 159–63 (1980).

14. White, A. Psychiatric study of patients with severe burn injuries. *British Medical Journal*, **284**, 465–67 (1982).

15. Culpan, R. & Davies, B. Psychiatric illness at a medical and a surgical outpatient clinic. *Comprehensive Psychiatry*, **1**, 228–35 (1960).

16. Goldberg, D. A psychiatric study of patients with diseases of the small intestine. *Gut*, **11**, 459–65 (1970).

17. Mayou, R. Psychological morbidity in a clinic for sexually transmitted disease. *British Journal of Venereal Diseases*, **51**, 57–60 (1975).

18. Vazquez-Barquero, J., Padierno Acero, J., Perra, C. & Ochotellio, A. The psychiatric manifestations of coronary pathology. *Psychological Medicine*, **15**, 585–96 (1985).

19. Farmer, C., Snowden, S. & Parsons, V. The prevalence of psychiatric illness among patients on home dialysis. *Psychological Medicine*, **9**, 509–514 (1979).

20. Byrne, P. Psychiatric morbidity in a gynaecology clinic. *British Journal of Psychiatry*, **144**, 28–34 (1984).

21. Brody, D. Physician recognition of behavioral, psychological and social aspects of medical care. *Archives of Internal Medicine*, **140**, 1286–89 (1980).

22. Pedder, J. & Goldberg, D. A survey by questionnaire of psychiatric disturbance in patients attending a VD clinic. *British Journal of Venereal Diseases*, **46**, 58–61 (1970).

23. Goldberg, D. & Blackwell, B. Psychiatric illness in general practice. *British Medical Journal*, **2**, 439–43 (1970).

24. Skuse, D. & Williams, P. Screening for psychiatric disorder in general practice. *Psychological Medicine*, **14**, 365–77 (1984).

25. Goldberg, D., Rickels, K., Downing, R., & Hesbacher, P. A comparison of 2 psychiatric screening tests. *British Journal of Psychiatry*, **129**, 61–67 (1976).

26. Hoeper, E., Nycz, G., Cleary, P., Regier, D. & Goldberg, I. Estimated prevalence of RDC mental disorder in primary medical care. *International Journal of Mental Health*, **8** (2), 6–15 (1979).

27. Spitzer, R. L. & Endicott, J. *Schedule for affective disorders and schizophrenia – Lifetime version.* New York, New York Department of Mental Hygiene, New York State Psychiatric Institute, Department of Biometrics Research, 1978.

28. Rogan, W. & Gladen, B. Estimating prevalence from the results of a screening test. *American Journal of Epidemiology*, **107**, 71–76 (1978).

29. Goldberg, D. Estimating the prevalence of psychiatric disorder from the results of a screening test. In J. K. Wing, P. Bebbington, & L. N. Robins (Eds.), *What is a case?* London, Grant McIntyre, 1981.

30. Marks, J., Goldberg, D.& Hillier, V. Determinants of the ability of general practitioners to detect psychiatric illness. *Psychological Medicine*, **9**, 337–53 (1979).

31. Nielsen, A. & Williams, T. Depression in ambulatory medical patients. *Archives of General Psychiatry*, **37**, 999–1004 (1980).

32. Chancellor, A., Mant, A. & Andrews, G. The general practitioner's identification and management of emotional disorders. *Australian Family Physician*, **6**, 1137–1143 (1977).

33. Goldberg, D. & Huxley, P. *Mental illness in the community.* London, Tavistock Publications, 1980.

34. Cooper, P., Gath, D., Rose, N. & Fieldsend, R. Psychological sequelae to elective sterilisation: A prospective study. *British Medical Journal*, **284**, 461–64 (1982).

35. Schmale, A. & Iker, H. Hopelessness as a predictor of cervical cancer. *Social Science and Medicine*, **5**, 95–100 (1971).

36. Murphy, E. & Brown, G. Life events, psychiatric disturbance and physical illnesses. *British Journal of Psychiatry*, **136**, 326–38 (1980).

37. Craig, T. K. J. Life stress and psychiatric disorder in the aetiology of abdominal pain. In G. W. Brown & T. O. Harris (Eds.), *Life events and illness.* New York, Guilford Press, 1986.

38. Whitlock, F. & Siskind, M. Depression and cancer: A follow-up study. *Psychological Medicine*, **9**, 747–52 (1979).

39. Greer, S. & Silberfarb, P. Psychological concomitants of cancer – current state of research. *Psychological Medicine*, **12**, 563–73 (1982).

40. Muhangi, J. Functional or organic psychosis. *African Medical Journal*, **3**, 319–26 (1972).

41. Maguire, G., Lee, E., Bevington, D., Kuchemann, C., Crabtree, R. & Cornell, C. Psychiatric problems the first year after mastectomy. *British Medical Journal*, **1**, 963–65 (1978).

42. Morris, T. Psychological adjustment to mastectomy. *Cancer Treatment Reviews*, **6**, 41–61 (1979).

43. Creed, F. Life events and appendicectomy. *Lancet*, **1**, 1381–85 (1981).

44. Kleinman, A. & Kleinman, J. Somatisation. The interconnections among culture, depressive experiences and the meaning of pain. In A. Kleinman & B. Good (Eds.), *Culture and depression*. Berkeley, CA: University of California Press, 1985.

45. Katon, W., Ries, R. & Kleinman, A. A prospective DSM-III study of consecutive somatisation patients. *Comprehensive Psychiatry*. In press.

46. Marsella, A. Depressive experience and disorder across cultures. In H. Trisandis & J. Draguns (Eds.), *Handbook of cross cultural psychiatry*. Vol. 8. Boston, Allyn & Bacon, 1979.

47. Racy, J. Somatisation in Saudi women. *British Journal of Psychiatry*, **137**, 212–16 (1980).

48. Bazzoui, W. Affective disorders in Iraq. *British Journal of Psychiatry*, **117**, 195–203 (1970).

49. Binitie, A. A factor-analytical study of depression across African and European cultures. *British Journal of Psychiatry*, **127**, 559–63 (1975).

50. Holmes, J. & Speight, A. The problem of non-organic illness in Tanzanian urban medical practice. *East African Medical Journal*, **52**, 225–36 (1975).

51. Sethi, B. Depression in India. *Journal of Social Psychology*, **91**, 3–13 (1973).

52. Kleinman, A. *Patients and healers in the context of culture*. Berkeley, University of California Press, 1980.

53. Cheung, F. Somatization among Chinese depressives in general practice. *International Journal of Psychiatry in Medicine*, **10**, 361–74 (1981).

54. Mezzich, J. & Raab, E. Depressive symptomatology across the Americas. *Archives of General Psychiatry*, **37**, 818–23 (1980).

55. Orley, J. H. & Wing, J. K. Psychiatric disorders in two African villages. *Archives of General Psychiatry*, **36**, 513–20 (1979).

56. Goldberg, D. Detection and assessment of emotional disorder in a primary care setting. *International Journal of Mental Health*, **8** (2), 30–48 (1979).

57. Bridges, K. & Goldberg, D. P. Somatic presentations of DSM-III psychiatric disorders in primary care. *Journal of Psychosomatic Research*, **29**, 563–69 (1985).

58. Beard, G. *A practical treatise on nervous exhaustion*. New York, William Wood & Co., 1880.

59. Kleinman, A. Neurasthenia and depression: A study of somatisation and culture in China. *Culture, Medicine and Psychiatry*, **6**, 117–90 (1982).

60. Katon, W., Kleinman, A. & Rosen, G. Depression and somatisation: A review. *American Journal of Medicine*, **72**, 241–47 (1982).

61. Nemiah, J. & Sifneos, P. Psychosomatic illness: a problem in communication. *Psychotherapy and Psychosomatics*, **18**, 335–40 (1970).

62. Rosen, G. Somatisation in family practice. *Journal of Family Practice*, **14**, 493–502 (1982).

63. Steinberg, H., Torem, M. & Saravay, S. An analysis of physicians' resistance to psychiatric consultations. *Archives of General Psychiatry*, **37**, 1007–1011 (1980).

64. Mezey, Z., & Kellett, J. Reasons against referral to a psychiatrist. *British Journal of Psychiatry*, **47**, 315–19 (1971).

65. Shepherd, M., Cooper, B., Brown, A. & Ralston, G. *Psychiatric illness in general practice.* London, Oxford University Press, 1966.

66. Johnson, D. Treatment of depression in general practice. *British Medical Journal,* **2**, 18–20 (1973).

67. Johnson, D. A study of the use of antidepressant medication in general practice. *British Journal of Psychiatry,* **125**, 186–92 (1974).

68. Rawnsley, K., Loudon, J. & Miles, M. Factors influencing the referral of patients to GP's. *British Journal of Preventive and Social Medicine,* **16**, 174–82 (1962).

69. World Health Organization. *Mental health: Report of the WHO Regional Expert Panel on Mental Health* (AFRO Report Series No. 7). Brazzaville, WHO Regional Office for Africa, 1979.

70. Hardy, T., Arango, M., Baltazar, J., Climent, C., Ibrahim, H., Ladrind Ignacio, L., Murthy, R. & Wig, N. Mental disorders in primary health care. *Psychological Medicine,* **10**, 231–41 (1980).

71. Murthy, R., Srinivasa. Mental health components in primary health care manuals: A review. *NIMHANS Journal,* **1**, 91–98 (1983).

72. Wig, N. & Murthy, R. S. *Manual for mental disorders for primary care.* Chandijarh, India, Persmelle Post Graduate Institute of Education, 1981.

73. Essex, B. & Gosling, H. An algorithmic method for management of mental health problems in developing countries. *British Journal of Psychiatry,* **143**, 451–59 (1983).

74. Johnstone, A. & Goldberg, D. Psychiatric screening in general practice. *Lancet,* **1**, 605–608 (1976).

75. Hoeper, E., Nycz, G., Kessler, L., Burke, J., & Pierce, W. The usefulness of screening for mental illness. *Lancet,* **1**, 33–36 (1984).

76. Bruhm, J., Wolf, S. & Philips, B. U. A psychosocial study of surviving male coronary patients and controls followed over 9 years. *Journal of Psychosomatic Research,* **15**, 305–313 (1971).

77. Querido, A. Forecast and follow-up. *British Journal of Preventive and Social Medicine,* **13**, 13–49 (1959).

78. Cay, E. L., Vetter, N. & Philip, A. E. Psychological status during recovery from an acute heart attack. *Journal of Psychosomatic Research,* **16**, 425–35 (1972).

79. Follette, W. & Cummings, N. Psychiatric services and medical utilisation. *Medical Care,* **5**, 25–35 (1967).

80. Goldberg, I., Krautz, G. & Locke, B. Effect of short term OP psychotherapy benefit on utilisation of medical services. *Medical Care,* **8**, 419–28 (1970).

81. Kogan, W., Thompson, D., Brown, J. & Newman, H. Impact of integration of mental health services and comprehensive medical care. *Medical Care,* **13**, 934–42 (1975).

8

The sociology of health care in developing countries

Debebar Banerji

A conceptual framework

The entire way of life of a community (i.e., its culture), including social and economic conditions, form a major category of factors that, along with biological and environmental components, determines the nature, scope, and distribution of health problems in that community. The culture of a community determines the health behaviour of the community and of its individual members, and the cultural response of the community to the health problems it confronts determines its health practices. All these elements form an interacting subsystem within the overall cultural system.

The health behaviour of the individual is closely linked to the way he or she perceives various health problems: what they actually mean to him or her, on the one hand, and, on the other, his or her access to various relevant institutions. For example, when a poverty-stricken agricultural labourer consults the village medicine-man for problems associated with his wife's pregnancy, he is not necessarily a prisoner of his 'traditional culture': he may lack the financial means for seeking the help of the specialist obstetrician in the nearby town.

This complex whole embracing the cultural perception and meaning of health problems and the health behaviour of individuals within the context of the available and accessible health institutions is termed *health culture* (1). Like any other cultural entity, health culture undergoes change. Endogenous innovations, cultural diffusion, and purposive interventions from without all bring change to the health culture of a community. This concept of health culture is central to an understanding of the sociology of health care in a country.

Thanks to a highly developed nervous system, the human being has been able to acquire considerable control over nature and over other living beings. But this very success in the struggle for existence has generated other categories of

The author is Professor and Chairman, Centre of Social Medicine & Community Health, Jawaharal Nehru University, New Delhi, 11067, India.

problems, chief among which are the exploitation of human beings by others of their species and the very rapid rate of growth of the earth's population. As a consequence of these problems, millions of human beings are still living under very adverse ecological conditions, which create a vicious circle for those who are subjected to them: such conditions are detrimental to people's health and, at the same time, reduce the power of the afflicted people to cope with the other vicissitudes confronting them.

Health problems and health practices within a community can be considered functions of the prevailing ecological conditions, which include cultural, social, and economic factors. Whenever human groups have succeeded in creating ecological conditions that are congenial for them, there has been considerable improvement in their health status, which then aids them in gaining access to much more potent tools for coping with the health problems that remain. The opposite situation prevails for human groups that are forced to continue living under adverse ecological conditions.

Sociological implications of the introduction of western medicine into developing countries

In the pre-industrial era, communities' health cultures developed in ways compatible with their overall mode of living. The more highly organized and refined a community's way of life, the more developed was its health culture – and vice versa; and since the mode of living at that stage in man's history was essentially rather 'simple', so was his health culture. The health practices that developed were the communities' response to the problems they encountered, though there was some diffusion of such practices among neighbouring communities.

Urbanization, the institution of slavery, mining activities, and warfare frequently caused disruption of this equilibrium and led to the formation of a new one, which often was unfavourable to the people. Nevertheless, because of the relatively small proportion of the population involved, and because the health culture was still very rudimentary in form, the impact of these factors on the total population was relatively slight.

The Industrial Revolution in European countries produced an extensive and far-reaching disruption in this equilibrium, affecting social, economic, and political relations in addition to the health culture. Many industrial workers were exposed to very adverse ecological conditions (2). Urbanization and industrialization also led to considerable erosion of people's capacity to cope with their own health problems. Technology became a very potent weapon in the hands of the rulers.

An even worse fate was in store for most of the people in the countries that were colonized by the industrialized countries. The establishment of health care services in colonized countries served the imperial policy of exploitation of these countries for the economic benefit of the colonial powers. Unlike in the industrial European countries, the health culture of the colonized countries went directly from a pre-industrial stage to a colonial one. This is a very important sociological issue in the study of health care in developing countries.

It is significant that the introduction of Western medicine sets very complex interactions in motion in a developing country. One major factor in these interactions is the very nature of Western medicine – its body of knowledge, its agencies for providing services of various kinds, its institutions for education, training, and research, and its corps of medical practitioners. These elements interact with the pre-existing health culture. Moreover, Western medicine has been associated with the far-reaching political, economic, and social changes that accompanied colonialism.

Changes in the health culture of India will serve as an illustration of how these factors can influence health care in a developing country.

A social analysis of health care services in India

There is substantial historical evidence that many centuries before Christ, Indian medicine had succeeded in making the momentous move from magico-religious to rational therapeutics (3. Pp. 48–51). Chattopadhaya has described the transition as follows:

> ... During [ancient Indian medicine's] creative period – the period of its transition from magico-religious to rationalistic therapeutics – the basic requirements of complete secularisation of their discipline led physicians to create a methodology of their own. Discarding scripture-orientation, they insist on the supreme importance of direct observation of natural phenomena and on the technique of a rational processing of the empirical data. They go even to the extent of claiming that the truth of any conclusion thus arrived at is to be tested ultimately by the criterion of practice .... Therapeutic power is conceived by them mainly in terms of the knowledge of [the] laws [inherent in nature]: the clearer the physicians's insight into these, the better is his prospect of regulating the interaction between body-matter and environmental matter, which determines disease and health. (Pp. 7–8)

This ushered in a wide range of theoretical and practical propositions, which attained an astonishingly high level of development. The unity of man and nature was the fundamental postulate of ancient Indian medicine.

There is also evidence that when certain political forces made Indian society hierarchical, the society sensed danger in everything that was conducive to the growth and development of sciences – e.g. secularism, the rational processing of empirical data, and the uninhibited search for laws of nature (3. P. 212).

> ... at least a section of the scientists tried to evade censorship by conceding to it, to add apparent conviction to its loyalty to the norm of orthodox piety. Special

chapters are added to [a] text for loudly proclaiming the theory of soul and its salvation. Fortunately, all these did not go to the fanatical extent of destroying what was once achieved by the ancient doctors.... What proved fatal for the creative development of Indian medicine [was] the gradual *erosion* among later doctors of the sense of total incompatibility between science and counter-ideology in the source-books of Indian medicine. They attached a sheer pragmatic value to the ancient drugs and decoctions and, practically oblivious of the marvellous science potentials or the theoretical achievements of the ancient doctors, go on dogmatically reiterating certain formulas as universal solvents of all pathogenic problems. (3. Pp. 425–26)

The history of medicine in India before the advent of the British is an account of encounters between the forces of obscurantism and the forces of reasoning. The decline in the social, economic, and political life of the country not only led to unfavourable shifts in the ecological balance but also created an environment in which obscurantism gained the upper hand. Perhaps the lowest point in this ecological crisis was reached during the decline of the Mughal Empire in the second half of the eighteenth century, a situation that set the stage for the British conquest of India. Even during this period the system of Indian medicine retained some remnants of its past heritage. For example, the surgeons of the British East India Company learned the art of rhinoplasty from Indian exponents of surgery (4. P. 500).

However, as a result of the colonial policy of shifting state patronage from the indigenous systems of medicine to the Western system, the already stagnant indigenous systems were caught in a vicious circle. Their very neglect accentuated their decline, which in turn made it increasingly difficult for the indigenous systems to compete with the highly favoured and rapidly flourishing Western system of medicine in capturing the imagination of the newly emerging educated elites of India. Thus, at a time when spectacular developments were taking place in the various branches of Western medicine, the indigenous systems became dominated by people with very limited competence, sometimes even by quacks and imposters; and the very scientific bases of these systems became almost totally eroded. The resulting vacuum was filled by a variety of superstitious practices and beliefs in supernatural powers and deities.

Hence, not only were the Indian masses denied the benefits of Western medical sciences by their colonial rulers but the total disruption of their way of life produced by colonialism caused a disruption of the practices they had developed in response to their health problems. Moreover, the colonial exploitation of the masses created adverse environmental conditions that further accentuated their health problems. The increased number of diseases generated by the disruption of the ecological balance, the breakdown in pre-existing health practices, and the denial of access to the Western system of medicine combined to worsen considerably the condition of the masses, making them even more vulnerable to exploitation (5, 6). At the same time, their rulers acquired additional strength by using the fast-developing knowledge of Western medicine to avoid illness and to obtain prompt and efficacious relief when they did fall ill. The health services thus served as a powerful weapon for solidifying colonial rule and, after India became independent, continued to be used to perpetuate an unjust economic and social order.

This analysis of the social, economic, and political determinants of the indigenous systems of medicine in India places them in a perspective quite different from the usual one. Unfortunately, most social scientists who have studied the health culture of the rural people of India have stressed their superstitious health beliefs and practices and have not paid adequate attention to the powerful social, economic, and political forces that were instrumental in causing the degeneration and decay of their health culture (7). Worse still, even in their descriptions of the existing situation they have betrayed a pronounced ethnocentric bias.

Marriott's study (8) of Western medicine in a northern Indian village is an example of the marked ethnocentric bias of Western scholars. He describes in detail how the only wage-earning son of a poor labourer did not accept the calcium lactate and shark-liver oil prescribed by a doctor (who, incidentally, was a white man and a missionary) for his tuberculosis and instead incurred debt to buy a preparation of honey and gold that had been made and guaranteed by an indigenous practitioner. On the other hand, a carefully designed study (9) of the social epidemiology of tuberculosis in the rural Tumkur district of Karnataka revealed that more than half of the victims of tuberculosis in the district who visited a government institution where Western medicine was practised were almost invariably dismissed with a bottle of useless cough medicine. Similar findings concerning villagers' failure to obtain effective Western medical care from health institutions are contained in an intensive study (10) of the overall health behaviour of rural populations in 19 villages located in eight states of India; and in a survey of a village in Tamil Nadu, Djurfeldt & Lindberg (11) also concluded that the people's felt needs for Western medicine were not being met by the relevant institutions.

After India gained its independence, the new political leaders made egalitarian pronouncements, but used essentially the machinery bequeathed them by the British (12). They promised to take active steps to make the benefits of health services available to the masses, particularly to the weaker segments (13). For this purpose, they also promised a revival and strengthening of the indigenous systems of medicine. In actual practice, however, they went on following the old colonial tradition of giving supremacy to the Western system. Urban areas continued to be given more attention than rural areas in the development of both curative and preventive health services (14). Community resources were made available for the establishment of a number of hospitals, many of which had the latest in sophisticated equipment for providing intensive care, open-heart surgery, brain surgery, and cancer therapy, following the model of the industrialized countries. The Western industrialized countries also served as a frame of reference for institutions for education, training, and research (15). Personnel in these sophisticated, urban-based institutions have remained heavily dependent on their counterparts in the industrialized countries, and the latter have actively encouraged such dependence by providing 'technical assistance' in the form of training, consultation, and 'cheap' textbooks (16).

The political leaders and the health administrators have sought social legitimacy for their actions by pointing to some not very relevant social, cultural, and psychological issues raised by social scientists. Value-laden issues such as modernization versus traditionalism and urban culture versus traditional folk culture have been used to justify the urban- and privilege-based health services in India (8, 17–19). It is claimed that the backward, superstition-ridden, uneducated villagers first have to be 'educated' by a corps of 'well-trained' health educators from the cities who can impart the virtues of 'modern' health services, which bear all the trappings of promotion of dependence and a profit orientation (7).

The elite-oriented services in India have followed the lead of the affluent countries, which actively promote dependence on health professionals (20), in their increasing tendency toward commercialization and professionalization of the health services and, in the process, have absorbed more and more of the country's health resources. The excessive preoccupation of the leadership with the urban health system has led to neglect of the rural health services. Not only has the rural health services system been starved of resources but, perhaps more important, the technical content of the services and the 'culture' and values of the personnel in the rural system have often been inimical to the needs of the rural population (7). Because of these factors, the rural health services can provide care for only a small fraction of the population – and even then, the accessible services are 'hand-me-downs', which educators and motivators are charged with making the people accept.

As early as 1920, the Indian National Congress (which spearheaded the independence movement in India) passed a resolution to the effect that, considering the popularity and generally accepted utility of the Ayurvedic and Unani systems of medicine, earnest efforts should be made to promote instruction and treatment in accordance with those systems (21). After India became independent, however, the indigenous systems of medicine were subjected to two contradictory pulls: their firm roots in Indian culture for centuries and their rich heritage invoked considerable admiration, even a certain degree of emotional attachment, from a large segment of the population; but long neglect of these systems of medicine had led to very sharp deterioration in their bodies of knowledge, their institutions for training and research, their pharmacopoeias and drug industry, and their corps of practitioners.

True to its 'soft state' approach (12), the political leadership of the country has paid lip service to the indigenous systems of medicine in order to gain popularity while, at the same time, vigorously expanding the Western system of medicine, which is much more in tune with its interests. Investment in the indigenous systems of medicine has been almost negligible compared with that in the Western system (22). A much more serious aspect of this approach is that, unlike in China, the indigenous systems of medicine have never been taken seriously by the political leadership: they are treated as stepchildren, and there are differences in the salaries of practitioners of the two systems, which are reflected in differences in the quality of the scholars who opt for the respective systems. Efforts to rediscover, through research, the lost heritage of indigenous systems of medicine, to get rid of the obscurantist elements that had crept into them, and to promote further growth and development of these systems have been very half-hearted and superficial (22). Efforts in relevant areas of education, training, and practice have been equally half-hearted (22).

Because of these developments, contrary to the prevailing 'belief', rural people have lost their enthusiasm for the indigenous systems of medicine. The intensive study of health behaviour in 19 villages referred to above (10) revealed that the response to major medical care problems was very much in favour of the Western (allopathic) system of medicine, irrespective of social, economic, or occupational considerations. Availability of such services and the ability of patients to meet their cost were the two major constraints.

On the whole, the dispensary of the primary health centres (PHCs) has projected a very unsatisfactory image. Because of this, and because of its limited capacity, the PHC has been unable to meet a very substantial proportion of the villagers' demands for health care. This enormous felt but unmet need for care has been the main motive force in the emergence of a large number of so-called registered medical practitioners (RMPs) or 'quacks'. The RMPs have, in effect, been created as a result of the inability of the PHC dispensary or other services staffed by qualified practitioners of Western medicine to meet the demand for medical care in the villages. It is worth noting that most RMPs use allopathic rather than Ayurvedic or Unani medicine. When they prove ineffective, villagers, depending on their economic status and the severity of their illness, actively seek help from government or private medical agencies in towns or cities.

Numerous instances of adoption of the healing practices of qualified or non-qualified practitioners of the different indigenous systems of medicine, of homeopathy, or of other, nonprofessional healers were observed in the village study (10). But only a very few of those suffering from major illnesses chose these practices and rejected accessible facilities in which Western-style medicine was practised. Usually people had recourse to the 'other' practices or to 'home remedies' (a) in conjunction with Western medicine, (b) after Western medicine had failed to give results, (c) when Western-type medical services were not accessible, or, most frequently, (d) when the illnesses were minor in nature.

The political leadership in India is now realizing that it is no longer possible to perpetuate the present social order without making some 'concessions' to the masses. Health services have apparently been singled out as an area for such concessions, on the presumption that, unlike sensitive areas such as land reforms, a minimum wage, and democratization, i.e. involvement of the people in their own governance, they will not pose a major threat to the social system. Indeed, the leaders who assumed political power in India in March 1977 by taking advantage of the people's resentment about the family-planning excesses of the previous months redeemed their election pledge and initiated a new programme based on village-level community health workers (23). And it is interesting that the government that followed, in 1980, did not dare to abolish the scheme of entrusting the people's health to local services. In fact, it issued, in 1982, a Statement on National Health Policy that called for 'involving the community in the identification of [its] health needs and priorities as well as in the implementation and management of health and related programmes' (16).

This is a most remarkable development, though it is obvious that the existing social structure and prevailing culture of the elite-oriented, professionalized health system are grossly incompatible with such a 'philosophy' and that this philosophy has already been greatly distorted by these forces (24). Nevertheless, this commitment of the political leadership to bypass the medical establishment and go directly to the people has created a very favourable setting for challenging the basic scientific, sociological, and economic premises of the earlier approach to the development of health services in India and for formulating an alternative approach.

At issue in formulating an alternative is not what should be the 'mix' of Western and indigenous systems of medicine in the health services of the country: the issue, essentially, is to offer an alternative that rectifies the distortions that have crept into the health services system because of the interplay of political, social, and economic forces. As Foster (25) has pointed out, it is particularly important to distinguish between the true clinical core of scientific (Western) medicine and the surrounding folk magic, customs, and faddism that are included in that system. The same principle applies to the indigenous systems of medicine: just as their neglect is undesirable, so is their romanticization, particularly in view of the degeneration that has set in within these systems because of political and social forces.

Health for and by the people

An alternative health services system should start with the people. Instead of fitting people into a predetermined framework, a health care system specially tailored to meet their needs must be designed. The technological elements should be consonant with relevant aspects of the pre-existing health behaviour, health institutions, and health care delivery agencies in the community, be compatible with the social and cultural setting, and be able to be implemented with the resources that can be made available for health purposes. In other words, people should not be 'educated' to discard the health measures they have adopted unless, taking into account *their* perception of the problems and the existing resource constraints, they can be convinced that an alternative technology will yield significantly greater benefits to them in terms of alleviation of the suffering caused by their health problems.

Some of the sociological dimensions of health care are brought into sharp focus by the cases described in the World Health Organization (WHO) publication *Health by the People* (26). In countries exemplified by China and Cuba, very positive efforts have been made to involve the entire population in the process of decision making as part of a nationwide political movement for bringing about radical social change. An alternative perspective for rural development and, as one of its components, an alternative health services system has developed as a logical corollary of this. In these countries the very process of achieving democratization of the political system led to serious questioning of the technological, social, and economic bases of the existing health services system.

In Tanzania, where serious attempts were being made to promote democratization at the grass-roots, the health services system inherited from colonial rulers was subjected to close examination. This led to a shift in allocation of resources from the cities to the rural areas, from curative to preventive services, and from an orientation toward service for the privileged class to one focusing on care of the underprivileged.

In every one of these cases, all sectors of the community, particularly its weaker elements, were actively involved in the shaping of an alternative primary health care system and in its implementation.

Significantly, in countries where the process of democratization has not made much headway, there is considerable hesitation, often even confusion, in designing alternative health services systems. The WHO publication describes two categories of such cases.

One is exemplified by two oil-rich countries, in both of which the political system had not allowed any change in the highly sophisticated, state-subsidized, curative services in urban areas, accessible largely to the privileged classes. Both of these countries, however, happened to have very dedicated leaders, in the persons of C. L. Gonzales, in Venezuela, and Majid Rehnama, in Iran. Despite stifling political constraints, they managed to achieve significant innovations in the rural health services of their countries. With the change of regime in Iran, most of the gains have been lost, proving that no lasting change is possible if it centres solely on charismatic personalities and lacks a solid base.

The other category is exemplified by Guatemala, India, and Indonesia. In all three countries the process of democratization has not reached the underprivileged and deprived segments of the population to any extent. Moreover, there has been a conspicuous lack of leadership in health care, which may explain why inspiration for alternatives was sought in the experiences of Christian missionary organizations. These experiences centred on programmes that had available to them resources that were disproportionately large for the very small populations served, plus workers fired by missionary zeal. These conditions are certainly not reproducible, and can by no means provide a model for designing alternative health care systems for rural populations in these countries.

The formation of alternative systems is essentially a political question. A crucial determinant of the nature of an alternative is whether the political system encourages oligarchical rule or actively promotes a change in the social order that enables the masses, particularly the underprivileged and the underserved, to participate in the affairs of their country (27).

The sociology of primary health care

Changes in the approaches of the World Health Organization to the health services development of its Member States during the past three decades and a half reflect changes particularly in developing countries. WHO policies are governed by its Member States through its World Health Assembly and its Executive Board, and developing countries now constitute an overwhelming majority of its members. Even if this were not the case, these countries would be the principal focus of WHO activities since their need for assistance is the most acute.

WHO started off with considerable enthusiasm for what have been referred to as 'vertical' programmes. These took the form of mass campaigns against individual health problems such as malaria (28), smallpox (29), tuberculosis (30), filariasis (31), leprosy (32), trachoma (33), schistosomiasis (34, 35), and yellow fever (36). These campaigns were designed according to a model consisting of a preparatory phase, an attack phase, a consolidation phase, and a maintenance phase. The approach was 'top-down', based on the expectation that technological interventions with weapons such as DDT spraying or the administration of penicillin, hetrazan, or dapsone would lead to the conquest of such dreaded diseases in 'underdeveloped' countries. It was assumed that these countries needed merely an effective 'technological fix' for their individual health problems.

When, after a decade and a half, WHO realized that such simple solutions did not work, it shifted its strategy to integration of mass campaigns against individual

188   *Debebar Banerji*

diseases into general health services (*37*). This basic shift in favour of integrated health services led to emphasis on the development of what were then termed the Basic Health Services (*38*. P. 69).

Yet another major shift in approach (in 1969) led to promotion of health planning (*39, 40*). First, it was health planning based on a more centralized concept. Later, the emphasis shifted to looking at health planning against the background of the actual conditions prevailing in specific countries. A 'Programme Systems Analysis' approach (*41, 42, 38*. P. 53) was followed by 'Country Health Programming' (*43, 44, 38*. Pp. 58–60), which, in turn, was succeeded by 'Country Health Planning'. Linking the entire health service system with the social and economic development of a country marked yet another phase (*45*).

Universal acceptance of the philosophy of primary health care at Alma Ata (*46*) by the countries of the world can be considered the climax of WHO's efforts at health services development. A major watershed, if not the most important one, in the history of medicine, the concept of primary health care involves virtually overturning the entire health services system of all countries in order to ensure that medical technology will subserve the community and that the distortions brought about by powerful market forces, undue professional dominance, iatrogenesis, and obsession with technological advances will be corrected. It advocates an intersectoral approach, integration of health services, and reorganization of the support structure so as to strengthen health work at the community level.

In the light of the perceptions of WHO Member States in WHO's early days, it is not surprising that the Organization should have embarked on a crusade against individual diseases through military-style mass campaigns. Why, then, did Member States go along with, if not actively promote, the various shifts that have culminated in acceptance of the primary health care approach?

It is possible to identify three factors that have contributed to this development. First, and perhaps most important, is the gradual increase in forces of democratization among the masses in the developing countries. The resulting pressures within some Member States impelled WHO to shift its approach. Second, headed by the Director-General himself, some thoughtful workers within the WHO Secretariat realized the need for change and used the Organization's forums to persuade member countries to undertake the changes it proposed (*46*). Finally, as a result of the momentum generated jointly by some Member States and the WHO Secretariat, other Member States were swept into the mainstream and adopted the new perspective proposed by WHO at Alma Ata. But obviously, the extent to which the primary health care approach is implemented in each country depends on the extent of the democratization of the people of that country and the readiness of its political leaders to respond to their democratic aspirations.

Summary and conclusions

The health care services of a community can be considered a cultural response of that community to its health problems, which are mediated by a complex inter-action of biological, environmental, cultural, social, and economic factors. Health services are closely linked with cultural perceptions of health problems, with their cultural meaning and the associated community behaviour; collectively, these elements are termed 'health culture'.

The concept of health culture provides a valuable framework for understanding the critical sociological forces involved in the introduction of Western medicine into a developing country. Western medicine is grafted onto cultural conditions in which it is essentially an alien element; it sets in motion complex interactions with the pre-existing health culture. Most important, the introduction of Western medi-cine has been associated with colonial exploitation, which caused considerable dis-ruption of ecological conditions for the vast majority of the population of the affected countries and limited access to health services largely to the colonial rulers and the most privileged sectors of the native gentry. Developments in India and in some other countries, the latter described by the World Health Organization, served to illustrate the health culture concept.

The conceptual framework outlined here may be used to assess the relevance of social science studies of health in developing countries, and may ultimately lead to an approach that will produce more meaningful studies of the sociological aspects of health care in those countries.

References

1. Banerji, D. *Poverty, class and health culture in India.* New Delhi, Prachi Prakashan, 1982. Vol. 1, p. 2.
2. Rosen, G. *History of public health.* New York, MD Publications, 1958. Pp. 131–90.
3. Chattopadhaya, D. P. *Science and society in ancient India.* Calcutta, Research India Publications, 1977.
4. Basham, A. L. *The wonder that was India.* London, Sidgwick and Jackson, 1954. P. 500.
5. Health Survey and Development Committee (Bhore Committee). *Report.* Vol. II. Delhi, Manager of Publications, 1946.
6. National Planning Committee, Sub-committee on National Health (Sokhey Com-mittee). *Report.* Bombay, Vora, 1948.
7. Banerji, D. Social and cultural foundations of health services systems of India. *Inquiry,* **12**(2), Suppl., pp. 70–85 (1975).
8. Marriot, M. Western medicine in a village of Northern India. In B. D. Paul (Ed.), *Health, culture and community.* New York, Russell Sage Foundation, 1955. Pp. 239–68.
9. Banerji, D. & Andersen, S. A sociological study of the awareness of symptoms suggestive of pulmonary tuberculosis. *Bulletin of the World Health Organization,* **29**, 665–83 (1963).

10. Banerji, D. Impact of rural health services on the health behaviour of rural populations in India: A preliminary communication. *Economic and Political Weekly*, **8**, 22 December, pp. 2261–68 (1973).

11. Djurfeldt, G., & Lindberg, S. *Pills against poverty: A study of the introduction of Western medicine in a Tamil village.* New Delhi, Oxford and ISH Publishers, 1975 (Scandinavian Institute of Asian Studies, Monograph Series, No. 23).

12. Myrdal, G. *Asian drama: An inquiry into the poverty of nations.* New York, Twentieth Century Fund, 1968. P. 243.

13. Borkar, G. *Health in independent India* (Rev. ed.). New Delhi, Ministry of Health, 1961. P. 11.

14. Indian Council of Social Science Research and Indian Council of Medical Research. *Health for all: All alternative strategy. Report of study group set up jointly by ICSSR and ICMR.* Pune, Indian Institute of Education, 1981. Pp. 3–10.

15. Government of India, Group on Medical Education and Support Manpower (Shrivastav Committee). *Health services and medical education: A programme for immediate action. Report.* New Delhi, Ministry of Health and Family Planning, 1975.

16. Government of India. *Statement on national health policy.* New Delhi, Ministry of Health and Family Welfare, 1982.

17. Carstairs, G. M. Medicine and faith in rural Rajasthan. In B. D. Paul (Ed.), *Health, culture and community.* New York, Russell Sage Foundation, 1955.

18. Hasan, K. A. *Cultural frontier of health in village India.* Bombay, Manektalas, 1967.

19. Khare, R. S. Folk medicine in a North Indian village. *Human Organization*, **22**, 36–40 (1963).

20. Ilich, I. *Medical nemesis: The expropriation of health.* Harmondsworth, Penguin, 1977.

21. Government of India, Committee on the Indigenous Systems of Medicine. *Report.* Vol. 1. New Delhi, Ministry of Health, 1948.

22. Government of India, Working Group on Health for All by 2000 A.D. *Report.* New Delhi, Ministry of Health and Family Welfare, 1981. Pp. 15–18.

23. Government of India. *Health care services in rural areas: Draft plan.* New Delhi, Ministry of Health and Family Welfare, 1977.

24. Government of India. *Health care services in rural areas: Revised plan.* New Delhi, Ministry of Health and Family Welfare, 1977.

25. Foster, G. M. *Problems of intercultural health programmes.* New York, Social Science Research Council, 1958.

26. Newell, K. W. *Health by the people.* Geneva, World Health Organization, 1975.

27. Banerji, D. Formulating an alternative rural health care system for India: Issues and perspectives. In J. P. Naik (Ed.), *An alternative system of health care service in India: Some proposals.* Bombay, Allied Publishers, 1977.

28. WHO Technical Report Series, No. 8, 1950 (Report on the third session of the Expert Committee on Malaria). Geneva, World Health Organization.

29. Basu, R. N., Jezek, Z. & Ward, N. A. *The eradication of smallpox from India* (WHO

Regional Publications, South-East Asia Series, No. 5). New Delhi, WHO Regional Office for South-East Asia, 1979. Pp. 309–312.

30. WHO Technical Report Series, No. 7, 1950 (Report on the fourth session of the Expert Committee on Tuberculosis). Geneva, World Health Organization.

31. WHO Technical Report Series, No. 87, 1954 (First report of the Expert Committee on Onchocerciasis). Geneva, World Health Organization.

32. WHO Technical Report Series, No. 71, 1953 (First report of the Expert Committee on Leprosy). Geneva, World Health Organization.

33. WHO Technical Report Series, No. 59, 1952 (First report of the Expert Committee on Trachoma). Geneva, World Health Organization.

34. WHO Technical Report Series, No. 17, 1950 (*Bilharziasis in Africa*: report on the first session of the Joint OIHP/WHO Study Group). Geneva, World Health Organization.

35. WHO Technical Report Series, No. 65, 1953 (First report of the Expert Committee on Bilharziasis). Geneva, World Health Organization.

36. WHO Technical Report Series, No. 19, 1950 (Report on the first session of the Yellow Fever Panel). Geneva, World Health Organization.

37. Gonzalez, C. L. *Mass campaigns and general health organization.* Geneva, World Health Organization, 1965 (Public Health Papers, No. 29).

38. World Health Organization, South-East Asia Regional Office. *A decade of development in South-East Asia, 1968–1977.* New Delhi, WHO Regional Office for South-East Asia, 1978.

39. WHO Technical Report Series, No. 350, 1967 (*National health planning in developing countries*: report of a WHO Expert Committee). Geneva, World Health Organization.

40. Hilleboe, H. E., Barkhuus, A. & Thomas, W. C., Jr. *Approaches to national health planning.* Geneva, World Health Organization, 1972 (Public Health Papers, No. 46).

41. Bainbridge, J. & Sapirie, S. *Health project management: A manual of procedures for formulating and implementing health projects.* Geneva, World Health Organization, 1974 (WHO Offset Publication, No. 12).

42. WHO Technical Report Series, No. 596, 1976 (*Application of systems analysis to health management*: report of a WHO Expert Committee). Geneva, World Health Organization.

43. WHO Official Records, No. 221, 1975. Geneva, World Health Organization. Pp. VII–VIII.

44. Mahler, H. Thirty-second World Health Assembly. *WHO Chronicle,* **33**(7–8), 245 (1979).

45. Abel-Smith, B., & Leiserson, A. *Poverty, development, and health policy.* Geneva, World Health Organization, 1978 (Public Health Papers, No. 69).

46. World Health Organization. *Primary health care: Report of the International Conference on Primary Health Care, Alma-Ata, USSR, Sept. 6–12, 1978.* Geneva, World Health Organization, 1978.

9

Population movements and health: global research needs

Patricia L. Rosenfield

People are on the move. In 1981, over 700 million passengers were carried by the world's airlines.[1] Many more people used less-monitored means of transportation: car, bus, train, boat, bicycle, donkey, foot. The reasons for these population movements are manifold — political, economic, social, medical — and they have been subjects of study for decades (1–4). The resulting social and economic consequences of population movements have also been topics of study and issues of traditional concern to policymakers.[2] Now, as growing numbers of people are introducing (and being introduced to) new elements in new environments, increasing heed is being paid to previously neglected consequence of population movements: health and associated changes in diseases.

My purpose here is to highlight research needs and opportunities in the area of health and population movements. Major research topics will be discussed and then summarized in a common conceptual framework. More detailed reviews of health-related issues associated with population movement, in both developed and developing countries, have been made by Velez (9) and Zarate.[3] Background documents and reports have been prepared for various meetings sponsored by the Pan American Health Organization, the World Health Organization, and other agencies, and will be discussed below.

Throughout this paper it is emphasized that the aim of research activities is to assist planners and managers in designing programmes to minimize the health-related hazards of population movements.

The author is Program Officer, Human Resources in Developing Countries, Carnegie Corporation of New York, 437 Madison Ave., New York, NY 10022. When this paper was written, she was Secretary, Scientific Working Group and Steering Committee on Social and Economic Research, UNDP/World Bank/WHO Special Programme for Research and Training in Tropical Diseases, Geneva, Switzerland.

This is a revision of a discussion paper presented at the 22nd Meeting of the Advisory Committee on Medical Research of the Pan American Health Organization, Mexico City, 7–9 July 1983.

Population movements and human health

Despite extensive discussion in the literature, there is no general agreement about terminology for research on population movements and human health. To try to establish some conformity – at least in usage of terms – the following definitions are proposed.

In this paper, the phrase *population movements* is used as the most general term covering all possible types of mobility and migration patterns. Movement out of or into an area with the intention to settle is called *migratrion*, a term that implies permanence. It is well established, however, that other types of movements are also common: people 'move' for very brief periods, e.g. to go to the marketplace; for slightly longer periods, e.g. to visit relatives overnight; or they may move seasonally for months for economic purposes, in response to labour demands. Such movements have been characterized as 'circulation patterns', implying that the people involved may return to their place of origin (*10*). It is recognized that more detailed terms may be necessary on a site-specific basis, but the following general terms broadly cover the possible movements over space and time. These terms are drawn largely from the work of Prothero (*11, 12*), who was perhaps the first to study, in a developing country context, people's movement behaviours and disease-specific health consequences.

Space	Time (example)	
Rural–rural	Migration:	planned (colonization projects)
Rural–urban		spontaneous (drought victim, refugees, squatters)
Urban–rural	Circulation:	daily (collecting firewood)
Urban–urban		periodic (pilgrimage)
		seasonal (harvesting)
		long-term (nomadic)

The physical hazards of moving – hazards that threaten both migrants and those already resident at the place of destination – have been described in relation to the development of chronic diseases and to the spread of infectious diseases (*13, 14*).

Zarate[4] refers to studies delineating various relationships between migration and chronic diseases:

> studies analysing the development of stomach cancer in Japanese who migrated to Hawaii;

> studies analysing similar development of stomach cancer in rural–urban migrants to Cali, Colombia;

> studies noting few adverse health affects of urban conditions (such as chronic bronchitis) among rural–urban migrants to Cracow, Poland.

Prothero (*11*), drawing on his work relating population movements in Africa to the transmission of infectious diseases, summarized the health consequences that may be faced at site of origin, in transit, and at new locations:

(1) exposure to diseases from movements through (and to) different ecological zones (e.g., malaria, trypanosomiasis, schistosomiasis, onchocerciasis);
(2) exposure to diseases from movements (or settlements) involving contacts between different groups of people (e.g. smallpox, poliomyelitis, AIDS);
(3) physical stress (e.g. fatigue, undernutrition/malnutrition); and
(4) psychological stress – problems of adjustment (and adaptation).

In areas where diseases such as malaria, trypanosomiasis, and schistosomiasis predominate, the role of population movements in disease transmission and control was an early concern in the organization of control efforts (*15*). For example, trypanosomiasis epidemics in Africa caused populations to flee, and such movements also served to introduce the disease into new areas (*16, 17*). In Sri Lanka, urban filariasis is rapidly becoming more frequent, even outpacing rural filariasis as the main filariasis problem in the country, because of the influx of rural migrants from filariasis areas to the urban periphery, where water supply and sanitation services are insufficient.[5]

As people move into newly created environments, they confront new diseases. This has been thoroughly documented with reference to water-resources-development projects throughout Asia, Africa, the Middle East, and Latin America (*18, 19*). While people are in the process of moving from one place to another, they may be exposed to new diseases. At the same time, people may also bring with them their own familiar diseases and create new problems at the sites through which they pass or at which they stay. For example, schistosomiasis-infected migrants who move by foot, animal, or motor vehicles may contaminate snail-infested water bodies at oases or rest stops along the way to their destination (*20*).[6] Those who travel by air or sea have contributed to bringing with them new insect vectors, such as mosquito vectors of malaria, dengue fever, and Japanese encephalitis. This has been documented in the case of countries in and around the Pacific Ocean, where, for example, in 1979 a tourist was responsible for an epidemic of Ross River virus in Fiji (*21*).

Moreover, people who move temporarily, e.g. for economic or religious reasons, often 'import' new diseases into or confront new diseases in their places of temporary residence. For example, between Rameswarem Island and nearby coastal areas in South India, both seasonal fishermen and pilgrims contribute 'to perpetuate malaria transmission in the island and in the coastal villages of the mainland' (*22*). Indeed, not only are diseases thus introduced and transmitted through population movements but drug-resistance in parasites or pesticide-resistance in vectors can be spread. This problem has complicated malaria control efforts in almost every part of the world (*23*).

Hence, a variety of health consequences, ranging from vector-borne diseases to mental health problems, can be identified and related to different types of population movement. This wide range of health effects indicates the complex task faced by planners in the development of appropriate health-care programmes (and other services as well) and suggests that an equally wide range of research efforts will be required.

Research in progress

A considerable amount of research has focused on the social, economic, and political factors that influence and result from population movements.[7] Although causes and consequences of ill health associated with population movements have been recognized on an historical basis, only recently has concerted effort been given to analyzing such problems in the specific context of developing countries (*9,24*).

Concern about the impacts in developing countries of the social, economic, and epidemiological factors associated with population movements led the Social Science and Medicine Subcommittee of the Pan American Health Organization's Advisory Committee on Medical Research to promote, through projects and meetings, the development of specific research activities. As a result, a project focusing on the relationship of malaria and seasonal worker movements is now under way in the Dominican Republic.[8] It is demonstrating that malaria is more prevalent where migrant workers are located than in the surrounding residential population. The complex of reasons for this is being examined in depth and is presumably related to living conditions and prior health conditions of the migrants.

Research is also under way to explore the impact of seasonal and labour-related movements between Burkina Faso and Côte d'Ivoire on trypanosomiasis transmission and control,[9] drawing heavily on related research done previously in the Onchocerciasis Control Programme in West Africa (*25*). These projects are exploring the linkages among (*a*) migrant and development variables of circulation, length of residence, and harvesting patterns; and (*b*) human exposure to the different tse-tse fly habitats, leading to different patterns of trypanosomiasis prevalence and incidence.

In Thailand the greatest risk facing the malaria-control programme has been the spread of drug-resistant malaria: 'The problem of the spread of drug-resistant strains of *P. falciparum* through the domestic movements of populations is a serious one in Thailand' (*26*. p. 102). The control programme staff have urged that, in addition to an increase in operational treatment and spraying activities, research be undertaken to determine how migration contributes to the spread of resistant strains. Such research should include the geographic range of such resistance, the development of specific epidemiological reporting systems, and 'evaluation of alternative or adapted technologies for different epidemiological, geographical and social situations; e.g. malaria checkpoints, personal protective measures, and careful follow-up of imported cases' (26. p. 105).

The development of the large-scale Mahaweli Scheme in Sri Lanka will attract thousands to an area of historic malaria endemicity. Research is under way to assess the present health status of this migrant population and the health impact of these settlements on the new agricultural environment (27).

The Federal Land Development Authority (FELDA) of the Government of Malaysia has taken what it calls a 'package deal approach' to assisting migrants that includes forest clearance, planting of major crops, village area development, settler selection and resettlement, infrastructural facilities, scheme management, and other processing, marketing, and social services.[10] To minimize adverse health consequences, FELDA emphasizes 'provision of adequate housing, education, transportation, water supply, health sanitation, family planning, recreational services'. FELDA staff have noticed increased awareness in the settlers of 'family health, nutrition and medical attention', and have suggested as research areas analyses of these changes in attitudes and the effectiveness of this approach in the development of future programmes.

In Latin America, problems of drug-resistant malaria, colonization of new territories, water-development projects, and agricultural development all serve to create new conditions for transmission of a variety of diseases.[11] However, in Brazil, a formal agreement has been reached between the Ministry of Health and the National Institute of Colonization and Agricultural Reform to study thoroughly in one region, on an experimental basis and before colonization, the health conditions of migrants and the new health conditions in the settlement areas, and to develop appropriate primary health facilities in advance.[12] Results of this innovative effort should be analysed to determine if the same approach might be feasible in other regions of Brazil and/or in other countries.

It is interesting to note that health conditions for migrant workers are also of concern in more-developed countries. A recent study (28) has documented the occurrence of diarrhoeal diseases and other infections directly linked to inadequate water supply and sanitation conditions in facilities for migrant farm workers in Salt Lake County, Utah, USA. For example, the rate of diarrhoea per 1000 clinic users was almost twenty times higher in the migrant population compared with the urban poor in the same county.

The social dislocations that result from seasonal or temporary movement should also be part of the analyses undertaken by health and disease-control planners. Short-term workers, who usually plan to stay only long enough to earn needed funds, but who may stay for years, as evidenced by the temporary workers and their families in the Gezira Scheme, Sudan (29), often do not have the opportunity to develop the sense of community that is being talked about now as the basis for the World Health Organization's global strategy of Health for All (30).[13] Organizing primary health care or disease-control activities within a community framework may not be realistic under these conditions; an alternative system of health-care delivery may need to be provided, at least until new social systems develop.

The impact of population movements on disease transmission and control in Latin America was reviewed at a meeting organized in Brazil in 1981 by the Superintendencia de Campanhas de Saude Publica, with support from the Pan American Health Organization, the UNDP/World Bank/WHO Special Programme for Research and Training in Tropical Diseases, and the World Health Organization (31). A fundamental point of consensus reached by the participants was that the purpose of research should be to improve the conditions for migrants and not to impose controls on people who wish to migrate:

> The main object of the activities, what the authorities' endeavour to control, should be the *disease*, not the *migrant*. When it is observed that migrants are spreading or causing health problems, the planner may be tempted to control migration. It must be remembered first and foremost, however, that the control of disease, as an objective, is consistent with all human values and is generally recognized as a human right, whereas the control of migration infringes on ethical and political principles of freedom of movement and human rights. This applies to everyone, including the sick. (*31*. P. 192)

This reaffirms historical concern about the freedom to move as 'expressed by an International Emigration conference in 1889: "We affirm the right of the individual to the fundamental liberty accorded to him by every civilized nation to come and go and dispose of his person and destinies as he pleases"' (*3*. P.9).

Research needs

Since 1981, several technical meetings have specifically addressed the relationship between population movements and transmission of disease. The participants at the above-mentioned meeting in Brazil, at later meetings in Hawaii in 1981, in Washington in 1982, and in Sri Lanka in 1983 have identified gaps in knowledge and understanding.[14] In 1985, the Panel of Experts on Environmental Management for Vector Control (PEEM) of the World Health Organization/United Nations Environmental Programme/Food and Agriculture Programme focused its annual technical discussions on the impact of population resettlement on vector-borne diseases. The panel noted: 'When human populations migrate to and from the project area as part of the development, changes in the eco-system and in vector borne diseases affecting the people may be complex and adverse'.[15] The par-

Table 1. *Research issues of particular relevance to population movements and health*

Social	Economic	Medical	Environmental	Operational
Attitudes (about health and health services)	Employment conditions	Genetic/immune status	Changes in vector breeding sites	Location and accessibility of services
Belief patterns (religious, disease-related)	Ownership of land and other assets	Drug resistance of parasites	Water-supply facility provision	Health education programmes
Behaviour patterns	Impact of disease (social and economic costs)	Chemical resistance of vectors	Sanitation conditions	Information to other sectors
Levels of knowledge about health and disease conditions and control measures	Access to facilities (e.g. time costs)	Introduction of 'foreign' pathogens and vectors	Housing conditions	Monitoring capabilities in areas of spontaneous movement or circulation
Levels of community development and organization	Agricultural patterns	Changes in health status of migrants and residents	Climatic changes	Response to demand for new services
Social contacts (at origin, in transit, at destination)	National and local political/economic structure	Nutritional levels and changes	Soil conditions	Services effectiveness in planned or spontaneous settlements
Impact of man-induced disasters		Psychological stress and adjustments (social concern also)	Impact of natural disasters	

ticipants indicated that research was needed in relation to preventive planning: 'There is a need for careful prediction of likely changes resulting from resettlement projects, including those associated with unplanned, spontaneous settlers'.[16]

The research recommendations made at these meetings, based on experiences and studies referred to above, can be categorized around five broad issues, summarized in the table: social, economic, environmental, medical, and operational. These research issues refer not only to studies of people who move, whether for short or long periods, but also to those who stay in the place of origin and those who reside in areas to which the migrants move. Although not indicated in the table, longitudinal studies of how conditions change as people's migratory status changes are also considered important. It must be emphasized that the topics listed in the table indicate only the range of questions to be answered in examining the health aspects of different types of movements. Specific research projects should be developed in the context of both the macro- and the micro-conditions of the research site.

The main objective of the recommended research studies is to assist in the planning and implementation of health programmes, either for primary health care or for disease control. As indicated in the table, the problems to be studied cover a wide range of disciplines; the research teams therefore need to be interdisciplinary. Researchers and research methods from sociology, anthropology, demography, geography, and economics as well as from epidemiology, parasitology, entomology, and ecology need to be integrated into the research efforts. Methods of analysis should combine (in ways yet to be generally agreed upon) qualitative and descriptive analytical techniques with the more quantitative methods of multivariate statistical analysis (9, 32, 33).[17] Thus, research in this area requires a practical orientation, drawing upon a variety of disciplines and research methods.

The needs listed in the table are drawn from a number of meetings held on this subject and are general in nature. They indicate the type of research questions that may be asked in a given situation. For a more thorough review, see Velez (9). It is expected that any research effort would be designed in the context of site-specific needs. The topics lister refer to all categories of migrants and residents.

A conceptual framework

'Studies of migrants are fraught with all the complexities and opportunities that the study of any social change entails' (34). As is apparent from the above discussion, studies on the health-related aspects of population movement are especially complex because of the need to examine simultaneously the social, economic, and environmental changes that interact with the health changes. In addition, the studies need to be carried out over a continuum of space and time in order to be able to assess the health consequences fully and to plan appropriate health measures. It is important to know the baseline conditions at the site from which people move, conditions along their path of movement, and conditions at the place where they settle. However, these conditions may change during the time people reside in an area; therefore, studies of health consequences need to be longitudinal.[18]

In Figure 1, a basic conceptual framework is proposed for studies of population movements and health. The baseline conditions of society, economy, and ecology, shaped as a result of historical processes, provide the background for these studies (see box 1). These baseline conditions determine the situation found in stable, steady-state communities prior to shifts in population or where the more limited circulatory movements might be part of daily life (e.g. going to the marketplace). The health status, social relations (including behaviour patterns), and economic status are outcomes of this stable situation (see box 2).

When the decision to move is made, whether for a long or a short term, the migrants pass through unfamiliar conditions that affect their health status, behaviour patterns, and social/economic situation. As strangers they find themselves in new physical environments with new diseases and without the social contacts to know where to find and how to use health-care facilities. This period of circulation or transit has its own particular set of health, social, and economic outcomes (see box 3).

Moreover, in the case of seasonal migrants, special services are unlikely to be developed unless, as occurs in some labour-camp situations, health services are provided by the company or government; usually, no special services are available. It is in this situation that serious health conditions can develop, adversely affecting both newcomers and long-term residents. Even if they return home after only a short stay away from their usual abode, the temporary migrants' social positions may be different, and their ability to cope with a familiar environment may be reduced or augmented, depending upon their experiences during periods of circulation. Demands for different services are likely to result.

Migrants who move permanently to new places face the same problems of adjusting to new conditions (see box 4). Such migrants, however, have time on their side (34). Depending on the services available, they may be immediately better or worse off. Over time, if a new community develops, some of the early problems may be alleviated, and a new equilibrium of health, social, and economic conditions may develop.[19]

This framework is only a preliminary one, and is suggested mainly as a means for organizing the varied research issues associated with studies of population movements and their health impacts. It is hoped that further development of such an analytical framework will contribute to the systematic growth of this area of health research.

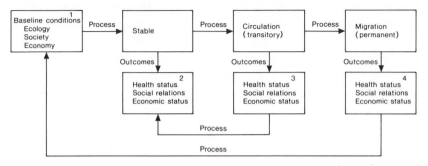

Fig. 1. Schematic representation of the relationship among baseline conditions, population movements, and outcome indicators. It should also be recognized that outcomes of these different processes of movement affect not only those who move but also those who stay behind and those who live in the areas through and to which people move.

Conclusion

As population movements within and between countries are increasing, so is public concern about associated health problems. Interdisciplinary research projects need to be promoted within the context of a conceptual framework, such as the one described here, in order to understand better the social, economic, and health consequences of population movements.[20]

Research projects need to be theoretically sound and, at the same time, practical in orientation, so as to yield results that can be easily incorporated into health and development programmes. To obtain practical results, research teams should be drawn not only from research institutions but also from ministries of health – and possibly from ministries concerned with economic development. Involving the eventual users of the research results from the initial stages of project design can help in identifying specific needs and developing operational solutions. Research will thus be action oriented from the start, and help to ensure that people affected by population movement can maintain, and eventually improve, their health.

Postscript

Since this paper was written, the complex of diseases known as acquired immune deficiency syndrome (AIDS) has appeared as a global problem, occasionally introduced into a country by tourists arriving on holiday or returning home, by truck drivers, or by migrant workers entering a country or returning home. In a few countries this has led to the imposition of quarantine regulations on those coming from reputedly high-risk countries, which limits the freedom of movement of travellers.

Although the mode of transmission of AIDS seems to be limited to sexual contacts, intraveneous drug use (through contaminated needles), and blood trans-

202   *Patricia L. Rosenfield*

fusion, there is still uncertainty about the relationship among frequency of exposure, quantity of the virus entering the bloodstream, and development of the disease. Consequently, even occasional contact must be considered a risk, which increases the likelihood that short-term movements can lead to disease transmission. An important area of research is systematic study of the relationship of short-term circulation patterns to the transmission of AIDS, with variables such as age, sex, neighbourhood, clan, class, income, and occupation being used to stratify the samples.

Notes

1. IATA World Transport Statistics, 1983 (telephone communication).
2. See references 1–8.
3. A. O. Zarate, Some consequences of internal migration: Migration and health. Invited paper, 44th Session of the International Statistical Institute, Madrid, Spain, 12–23 September 1983.
4. Ibid., pp. 3–5.
5. Dr. L. Mendis, Superintendent, Anti-Filarial Campaign, Sri Lanka. Personal communication, 1983.
6. F. H. Meskal, Vector-borne diseases related to labour movement and arrangements for their control (*PMO/PE/WP/85.4*). Paper given at Fifth Annual Meeting, Joint WHO/FAO/UNEP Panel of Experts on Environmental Management for Vector control, Bangkok, 7–11 October 1985.
7. See, for example, research supported by the International Development Research Centre, Ottawa, Canada; International Labour Office, Geneva, Switzerland; the Population Council, New York, USA. A good review is provided by Population Information Program: Migration, population growth and development. *Population Report*, series M, No. 7, September–October 1983. Although not discussed here, there is also increasing interest in documenting the experiences of international migration and Third World development by the International Committee for Cooperation in National Research in Demography (ICRED), Paris, and the Intergovernmental committee on Migration (ICM), Geneva.
8. D. Cury et al., Economic and social factors related with malaria in the Dominican Republic, project ID.810060. Ongoing project supported by UNDP/World Bank/WHO special Programme for Research and Training in Tropical Diseases, WHO, Geneva, Switzerland, 1981.
9. J. P. Hervouet, Systèmes d'occupation du sol, conditions sociales et transmission de la trypanosomiase, project ID.800079. Ongoing project supported by UNDP/World Bank/WHO Special Programme for Research and Training in Tropical Diseases. World Health Organization, Geneva, 1980.
10. Z. Mohammad, FELDA – A study in population movement and its impact on the strategies and patterns of human settlement and development. Unpublished material prepared for the Workshop on Human Population Movements, see note 14.

11. P. L. Castellanos, H. Corderio, S. Franco Agudelo, L. Lafontant, F. Paulino Mencia, E. Vanzie, *et al.*, Projecto de investigación sobre migraciones y enfermedades tropicales, unidad de promoción y coordinación de investigación. Washington, DC, OPS, 1982.

12. Dr. J. Fiusa Lima, Superintendent, SUCAM, Brazil. Personal communication, 1982.

13. Dr. J. Najera, Director, Malaria Action Programme, World Health Organization. Personal communication, 1983.

14. . East–West Center, Migration and adaptation among Asia–Pacific populations. Honolulu, Hawaii, August 1981 ; Organizacion Panamericana de la Salud (OPS), informal consultation on Migration and Tropical Diseases, Washington, DC, December 1982; M. Fernando (Ed.), *Proceedings of the Workshop on Human Population Movements and Their Impact on Tropical Disease Transmission and Control.* Peradeniya, Sri Lanka, 28 January–1 February 1983; S. Coulibaly, organizer, 1985, Patterns of settlement and their demographic implications. Session F–10, International Population Conference, International Union for the Scientific Study of Population, Florence, Italy, 5–12 June 1985.

15. WHO/UNEP/FAO Panel of Experts on Environmental Management for Vector Control, Report of technical discussions on the environmental impact of population resettlement and its effect on vector-borne diseases (*VBC/85.5*). World Health Organization, Geneva, 1985. P. 42.

16. Ibid., p. 44.

17. P. L. Rosenfield & P. J. Gestrin, Socio-economic analysis of impact of water projects on schistosomiasis. Unpublished report to Agency for International Development, Office of Health, Washington, DC, 1879. Pp. 30–45 ; R. E. Bilsborrow, Surveys of internal migration in low-income countries: The need for and content of community-level variables. Report to World Employment Programme, International Labour Office, Geneva, 1981. 63 pp.

18. A major recommendation made at the Workshop on Human Population Movements (op. cit.) and the WHO/UNEP/FAO meeting (op. cit.).

19. As indicated in the FELDA experience, op. cit., note 10.

20. Specifically for migration and develop studies, a similar approach to developing a conceptual framework is reported on by R. C. Jones & L. A. Brown, Cross-national tests of a third-world development–migration paradigm: with particular attention to Venezuela. *Socio-Economic Planning Science,* **79 (5)**, 357–61 (1985).

References

1. Milbank Memorial Fund. *Post war problems of migration.* New York, 1947.
2. Milbank Memorial Fund. *Selected studies of migration since World War II.* New York, 1958.
3. Thomas, B. *International migration and economic development.* Paris, UNESCO, 1961.
4. Mangalam, J. J. *Human migration: A guide to migration literature in English 1955–1966.* Lexington, University of Kentucky Press, 1968.

204   *Patricia L. Rosenfield*

5. Adepoju, A. Migration and socio–economic change in Africa. *International Social Science Journal,* **31** (2), 207–225 (1979).
6. Peek, P., & Standing, G. *State policies and migration* (World Employment Programme, International Labour Office). London, Croom Helm, 1982.
7. Castro, M., Neto, E., da Souza, M. D., Grabois, G. P. & Fraenkel, L. M. *Migration in Brazil: Approaches to analysis and policy design* (World Employment Programme, International Labour Office). Liège, Ordina Editions, 1978.
8. Glissant, E. (Ed.) Migrants: Between two worlds. *The Courier* (Pris, UNESCO), September 1985.
9. Velez, C. Migration and health: A literature review with emphasis on tropical diseases. In M. Fernando (Ed.), *Proceedings of the Workshop in Human Population Movements and Their Impact on Tropical Disease Transmission and Control.* Sri Lanka, Peradeniya, 28 January–1 February 1983. Pp. 153–76.
10. Prothero, R. M., & Chapman, M. *Circulation in Third World countries.* London, Routledge & Kegan Paul, 1985.
11. Prothero, R. M. Disease mobility: A neglected factor in epidemiology. *International Journal of Epidemiology,* **6** (3), 259–67 (1977).
12. Prothero, R. M. Population movements and problems of malaria eradication in Africa. *Bulletin of the World Health Organisation,* **24**, 405–25 (1961).
13. Wolstenhome, G. E. W. & O'Connor, M. *Immigration: medical and social aspects* (Ciba Foundation Report). London, J. & A. Churchill, Ltd., 1966.
14. Velemirovic, B. Forgotten people – Health of migrants. *Bulletin of the Pan American Health Organization,* **13** (1), 66–85 (1979).
15. *WHO Technical Report Series,* No. 123, 1957 (Sixth report of the WHO Expert Committee on Malaria). Geneva, World Health Organization. Pp. 59–63.
16. Prothero, R. M. Population mobility and Trypanosomiasis in Africa. *Bulletin of the World Health Organization,* **28**, 615–26 (1963).
17. Adekolu–John, E. O. The Significance of migrant Fulani for human trypanosomiasis in Kainji Lake area of Nigeria. *Tropical Geographical Medicine,* **30** (3), 285–93 (1978).
18. Hunter, J. M., Rey, L. & Scott, D. Man-made lakes and man-made diseases: Towards a policy resolution. *Social Science and Medicine,* **16**, (11), 1127–45 (1982).
19. Stock, R. Disease and development, or The underdevelopment of health: A critical review of geographical perspectives on African health problems. *Social Science and Medicine,* **23** (7), 689–700 (1986).
20. Kloos, H., Lemma, A., Kirub, B., Gebre, A., Mazengia, B., Feleke, G. & de Sole, G. Intestinal parasitism in migrant farm labour populations in irrigation schemes in the Awash Valley, Ethiopia, and in major labour source areas. *Ethiopian Medical Journal,* **18**, 53–62 (1980).
21. Self, L. S. Diseases associated with international travel. *Yonsei Reports on Tropical Medicine,* **15** (1), 65–69 (1984).
22. Rajagopalan, P. K., Jambulingam, P., Sabesan, S., Krishnamoorthy, K., Rajendran, S., Gunasekaran, K. & Kumar, N. Pradeep. Population movement and malaria

persistence in Rameswarem Island. *Social Science and Medicine,* **23** (7), 589–700 (1986).

23. Ray, A. P. The problem of dissemination of drug resistant falciparum malaria through population movement. In M. Fernando (Ed.), *Proceedings of the Workshop on Human Population Movements and Their Impact on Tropical Disease Transmission and Control.* Sri Lanka, Peradeniya, 28 January–1 February 1983. Pp. 117–23.

24. Van Ginnekan, J. D. & Muller, A. S. (Eds.) *Maternal and child health in rural Kenya: An epidemiological study.* London, Croom Helm, 1984.

25. Proust, A., Hervouet, J.–P., & Thylefors, B. Les niveaux d'endémicité dans l'onchocercose. *Bulletin of the World Health Organization,* **57**, 655–62 (1979).

26. Pinichpongse, S. & Doberstyn, B. The role of population migration in the spread of drug-resistant falciparum strains in Thailand. In M. Fernando (Ed.), *Proceedings of the Workshop on Human Population Movements and Their Impact on Tropical Disease Transmission and Control.* Sri Lanka, Peradeniya, 1984. Pp. 102, 105.

27. Wijesundera, M. Mahawali development and environmental health in Sri Lanka. In M. Fernando (Ed.), *Proceedings of the Workshop on Human Population Movements and Their Impact on Tropical Disease Transmission and Control.* Sri Lanka, Peradeniya, 1984. Pp. 177–80.

28. Arabab, D. M. & Weidner, B. L. Infectious diseases and field water supply and sanitation among migrant farm workers. *American Journal of Public Health,* **76** (6) 694–95 (1986).

29. Amin, M. Human population movements and their impact on transmission and control of schistosomiasis in irrigation schemes in the Sudan. In M. Fernando (Ed.), *Proceedings of the Workshop on Human Population Movements and Their Impact on Tropical Disease Transmission and Control.* Sri Lanka, Peradeniya, 1984. Pp. 1–4.

30. *Global strategy for health for all by the year 2000.* Geneva, World Health Organization, 1981 ('Health for All' Series, No. 3).

31. Ministerio da Saude and Superintendencia de Campanhas de Saude Publica (SUCAM). *Doenças e Migraçao Humana* Brasilia, Centro de Documentaçao do Ministerio da Saude, 1982 (Serie: Reunioes e conferéncias 1).

32. Verhasselt, Y. The contribution and future development of spatial epidemiology. *Social Science and Medicine,* **15A**, 333–35 (1981).

33. Van Ginneken, J. K., Omondi–Odiambo & Muller, A. S. Mobility patterns in a rural area of Machakos District, Kenya, in 1974–1980. *Tidjschrift Voor Econ. en Soc. Geografie,* **77** (22), 82–91 (1986).

34. Wessen, A. F. Migrant studies and epidemiological research. *Israel Journal Medical Sciences,* **7** (12), 1590 (1971).

10

Health and behaviour: a worldwide perspective

David Hamburg and Norman Sartorius

The health of the world is much more closely related to behaviour than we understood even a decade ago. Modern science and technology have made powerful contributions to knowledge of how to meet the basic adaptive needs for food, water, shelter, and other essentials for survival and reproduction. Yet we have been killing ourselves: inadvertently for the most part, knowingly to some extent, and regretfully – but killing ourselves none the less.

The heaviest burden of illness today is related to individual and group behaviour. It is reliably estimated that, in the United States, 50% of mortality from the ten leading causes of death can be traced to behaviour such as smoking, drinking, and eating inappropriate foods. Numerous other behaviours are also highly relevant to health and disease, both mental and physical, of the individual and those around him (e.g. violence and suicide).

The health problems of the developing world are no less related to behaviour, involved not only in mental illness but also in nutrition, sanitation, family planning, and accident prevention. The life-style factors identified as relevant in developed countries also affect developing countries. For example, smoking, which is a major cause of both cardiovascular disease and cancer and a contributor to many other chronic illnesses, and alcohol use and abuse, which are directly or indirectly involved in a number of illnesses and impairments, are on the rise in developing countries; they both dramatically illustrate how significant the contribution of behaviour is to the modern burden of illness.

Cigarette-smoking is the single most important environmental factor contributing to early death in the more developed countries. There are several lines of evidence that cigarette-smoking actually has a causal role in heart disease, cancer

Dr Hamburg is President, Carnegie Corporation of New York, 437 Madison Avenue, New York, NY 10022. Dr Sartorius is Director, Division of Mental Health, World Health Organization, Geneva, Switzerland.

206

(of the lungs, pancreas, esophagus, larynx, throat, and mouth), and respiratory disease (chronic obstructive lung disease, bronchitis, and emphysema). The effect depends on the dose: greater morbidity and mortality occur with more cigarettes smoked, higher tar and nicotine content, greater inhalation of cigarette smoke, and earlier age at initiation of smoking. Risk is reduced with quitting, but it may take years to return to the risk levels of people who have never smoked. Cigarette-smoking is even dangerous to the unborn child: a mother's smoking during pregnancy doubles the risk that she will have a low-birth-weight infant. Women who smoke during pregnancy also are at greater risk of serious complications in terms of their own health.

Alcohol abuse probably constitutes the most serious worldwide drug problem, affecting many millions of adult problem drinkers, their family members, and innocent bystanders who become the victims of alcohol-related accidents and violence. The misuse of alcohol is a factor in more than 10% of all deaths in most developed nations, and constitutes one of the main causes, worldwide, of work loss and family disruption. Heavy drinking is an important causal factor in damage to the liver and brain and in some cancers. As with smoking, alcohol use during pregnancy tends to be damaging to the foetus.

The burden of illness affecting a population can be measured in various ways, for example, by death rates caused by a particular factor, prevalence of a disease, inpatient days, days lost from work, limitation in the performance of activities, effects on quality of life, economic costs, and potential years of life lost (measuring from age at death to average life expectancy). Although each measure reflects a different aspect of the burden of illness, they all converge on the great extent to which strongly behaviour-related conditions figure in the burden of illness.

It is difficult to imagine a single publication that could comprehensively cover the relationships among health, behaviour, and disease. For this book it was therefore necessary to make a choice and to concentrate on perspectives that have received less emphasis in recent relevant literature. Making this selection was made easier by the fact that several important publications in recent years have addressed topics that would otherwise have to be discussed here (see, for example, *1.* Hamburg and associates, 1982).

There was, however, another factor that made the choice of perspectives presented here easier: the availability of information obtained in the course of implementation of the World Health Organization's programme on biobehavioural sciences and health. This programme was launched in 1980, following a recommendation made to the Director-General of the World Health Organization (WHO) by the Global Advisory Committee on Medical Research. In response the Director-General established a Scientific Planning Group on the Expanded Programme of Research and Training in Biobehavioural Sciences and Mental

Health, under the chairmanship of David Hamburg. The group reviewed previous WHO work, the scientific literature, and the information available through the WHO mental health programme.

The themes that emerged from this review and the group's discussions can be summarized as follows (WHO, 1982)[1]:

1. In developing countries, as in developed ones, health and behaviour are indivisible. Individual and community patterns of water use, hygiene, nutrition, alcohol and other drug use, and reproductive behaviour – to cite but a few relevant factors – directly affect health, for better or for worse.

2. The tightly focused, categorical approach of WHO's other expanded research programmes (on tropical diseases, human reproduction, and diarrhoeal diseases) is difficult to adapt to the area of mental health and biobehavioural science because no one type of behaviour stands out as the single most significant threat to health in developing countries.

3. An important precursor for an expanded research programme is a systematic assessment of the burden of illness that is attributable to psychosocial factors. An accurate overview of the scope of the problem, however, is vital to generating research interest and support.

4. High priority should be given to epidemiological research efforts aimed at pinpointing behaviour-related health problems in specific communities, cultures, countries, and regions. To conduct such research, rapid, culture-sensitive assessment techniques of 'community diagnosis' are needed.

5. Despite the immense cultural variability that makes it difficult to devise effective means of influencing health-relevant behaviour, certain basic principles – such as principles of learning – can be applied universally.

6. A central question to be addressed is common to developed and developing countries alike: how to present the issues in a way that will arouse and sustain the motivation of individuals and communities to adopt appropriate behaviours. It is important to identify programmes and practitioners who have succeeded and to analyze elements of their success that may be transferable, with appropriate modification, to other situations and cultures.

7. Political obstacles are more likely to arise in the sphere of mental health and biobehavioural research than in the other WHO expanded research programmes. These need to be anticipated and weighed in the selection of foci for the programme.

8. The development of a research infrastructure in developing nations is a key objective for the proposed WHO programme. Sustained collaborative arrangements with institutions in developed countries can be helpful in this regard.

9. In both developed and developing nations, there is a need to encourage far greater cooperation and collaboration between biomedical and behavioural scientists.

10. WHO should count on existing institutions in the developing countries,

rather than seek to establish new ones, in conducting its expanded programme in mental health and biobehavioural science. Logical candidates include: (*a*) existing units already involved in psychosocial research, (*b*) strong medical research units that currently lack behavioural research components, (*c*) excellent clinical units now lacking such research capability, and (*d*) research or clinical units in institutional settings where research is respected and supported.

11. Behavioural scientists already contribute to many WHO programmes, for example those dealing with human reproduction and child and family health. However, often these scientists work in isolation. There would be considerable advantages in developing a programme of research and training in biobehavioural sciences and mental health that would facilitate linkage among programmes and make the pool of expertise more easily available for consultation by a variety of governmental and non-governmental agencies.

12. Existing centres in developing countries, particularly if strengthened, might provide a useful focus for the kind of mental health and biobehavioural science research that is needed. These centres could also serve regional functions.

13. Problems of particular interest to a variety of developing countries include: community participation and motivation for primary health care; nutritional concerns, including the effects of changes in breast-feeding customs; child neglect, abuse, and understimulation; effects on mental and physical health of changes in family structure that occur with increased industrialization, migration, and uprooting; ways of changing hygienic practices related to drinking-water supply and sanitation; issues related to family planning; the effects of mass migration (both within countries and across countries) and of other major social changes on general health, family structure, and psychological state of individuals and social groups.

14. The Expanded Programme of Research and Training on Biobehavioural Sciences and Mental Health logically complements, and is integrated with, the mental health programme of the Organization. However, although directly related to the latter programme's objectives, it adds specific emphasis to a set of concerns and therefore deserves new consideration and support.

The planning group also defined two main priorities for action: first, strengthening research capacity within the developing countries; and, second, initiation and conduct of research in three major areas of investigation − (*a*) adaptation to rapid sociotechnical change; (*b*) control of alcohol problems, with particular emphasis on prevention in adolescence; and (*c*) promotion of child and family health through application of biobehavioural principles in primary health care.

Subsequently, task forces were established to deal with each of the three areas of investigation (WHO, 1983, 1984 a, b). They produced a research agenda for each of them and helped to launch a series of projects in different parts of the world. At the same time, efforts to establish or strengthen institutions that could undertake research on the relationship of health and behaviour continued, supported, *inter alia*, by an extensive programme of information collection and dissemination.

Time has clearly confirmed the wisdom of the planning group's recommendations. The social context of health and the psychosocial aspects of the development of children and adolescents have been receiving increased emphasis, in both political and scientific circles. Problems related to substance abuse have become a major concern to developed and developing countries.

Awareness of the need to develop techniques and organizational arrangements to deal with the mental health problems encountered in primary health-care settings has grown dramatically and the evidence that, in both developing and developed countries, as many as 15 % to 20 % of all contacts with medical services are occasioned by psychosocial problems has become more widely familiar; new studies, often aiming to disprove this finding, have invariably wound up confirming it.

These three topics – the social context of health (papers by Häfner & Welz, Banerji, and Rosenfield), the development of children and adolescents (papers by Graham, Hamburg, and Wachs), and mental health in general health care (the paper by Goldberg) – thus seemed to deserve priority in the selection of perspectives for inclusion in this volume.

Formidable obstacles to wider use of a psychosocial approach to health care are often the attitudes of health decision-makers who, because of training and other reasons, adhere to the biomedical model in the organization of health care to such an extent that they exclude any other way of viewing public health action. It was therefore important to add another perspective to this volume: a perspective which can illustrate psychosocial aspects of a 'nonpsychological' topic. The proper use of food and relevant nutritional programmes seemed to be well suited for this purpose, and a chapter discussing psychosocial factors affecting nutrition and food programmes was therefore added to the other three topics.

What follows in this introduction are the editors' comments on some of these themes. They should be considered in conjunction with the material presented in the chapters in which these themes are considered in depth.

Attachment, social support networks, and health

In modern times, the fundamental human propensity for attachment to other human beings is expressed in a largely unprecedented sociotechnical context – a world being rapidly transformed by the impact of science and technology. Mass media have a greater influence than ever before.

In advanced industrial societies, especially those characterized by high geographic mobility, the family is often so scattered that relations among its members are often drastically changed from traditional patterns. Separation and divorce have increased sharply in this century. In some developed countries, single-person households make up as many as one-third of all households in towns.

Very large social units engendered by the needs of industrial production have led to the rapid growth of immense cities. Such large entities tend to foster impersonal relations and add complexity to the attainment of close human relations. They also make it difficult to sustain the unity of purpose of small groups and the sense of community in which individuals share a strong mutual support ethos.

The recent body of research on the relationships among human attachments, illness, and mortality provides evidence, even when all known risk factors are statistically controlled, that people whose human attachments are weak are more vulnerable to illness and early death. Evidently, social support systems can buffer stressful experiences. Such networks also can influence the use of health services and adherence to preventive or therapeutic regimens, e.g. efforts to stop smoking. Social support systems offer opportunities to learn coping skills that help people maintain self-esteem, foster human relationships, and prepare for future tasks.

Observations of the beneficial effects of such systems have stimulated interest in social support networks on a worldwide basis, especially in circumstances of major transition and rapidly changing societies. They are of special significance in relation to the factors influencing healthy development during childhood and adolescence in contemporary societies. Currently, much innovative effort and some research are being devoted to strengthening social support networks where natural ones are weak.

A developmental perspective on health and behaviour

What we do early in life lays the foundation for all the rest, and can provide the basis for a long, healthy, life span. Early preventive intervention, when successful, is the most cost-effective. Worldwide, more than ten million children die each year of preventable diseases – it is as though a jumbo jet carrying several hundred children crashed several times each hour throughout the year.

Health and education are closely linked in the development of vigorous, skillful, adaptable young people. Investments in health and education can be guided by research in biomedical and behavioural sciences in ways likely to prevent much of the damage now being done to children and adolescents.

Although many causes underlie the developmental problems of the young, the most profound and pervasive factor is poverty. Almost every form of childhood damage is more prevalent among the poor – from increased infant mortality, gross malnutrition, recurrent and untreated health problems, and child abuse to educational disability, low achievement, early pregnancy, alcohol and drug abuse, dropping out of school, and failure to become economically self-sufficient.

Although poverty is a powerful factor in damage to children and adolescents, adequate income and high social status provide no assurance of healthy development. Alcohol and drug abuse, accidents, suicides, many health problems, and educational difficulties are plentiful in middleclass and highly privileged populations as well.

What can we do? During the past decade, careful inquiry in the biomedical and behavioural sciences has made it possible to learn about ways of preventing damage to children and adolescents. Prenatal care, prolonged breast-feeding, adequate nutrition, immunization, oral rehydration, antibiotics, early education, community-based education initiatives, and social support networks for health and education are among the effective interventions that have worldwide significance.

Two key indicators of the general condition of a society – not just in health but in education and the social environment as well – are infant mortality rates and maternal mortality rates. These measures are also proxies of more widespread troubles afflicting mothers and children in developing nations – and in poor communities everywhere. Young men and children are especially at risk of ill health and premature death in poor areas because of particular vulnerability during specific phases of the life span – those related to child-bearing in women, and the surge of growth and development in prenatal life and early childhood.

How many infants die before the age of 12 months per 1000 born? African countries have rates ranging from about 63 to 175 deaths per 1000 live births. In contrast, infant mortality rates in developed nations tend to be in the range of six to 12. Similarly, half a million women die in developing countries every year because of fertility-related conditions. In sub-Saharan Africa, maternal mortality rates range from two to six per 1000 births – 100 to 300 times the Western European rates. In rural Bangladesh, maternal mortality recently accounted for 57% of deaths of women aged 15 to 19 years old and 43% of deaths of women aged 20 to 29. When the mother dies, the health and welfare of the whole family are seriously jeopardized.

Mothers, children, and adolescents make up three-quarters of the populations of the developing countries. By reaching mothers with primary health care and by introducing health-promoting behavioural change – including, for example, family planning, higher literacy, and nutrition and other health education – the mother, as the primary caretaker, improves the status of the entire family. Most of the causes of death and severe disability among mothers and children are related to behavioural factors and are preventable at low cost.

Throughout the world, babies born too small for their gestational age are concentrated in poor, disadvantaged communities and among early-adolescent mothers. Low birth weight is a high risk factor for infant mortality and a source of lifelong problems, physical and mental, in the survivors. Several behavioural factors increase the risk of low birth weight: smoking, abuse of alcohol and other substances during pregnancy, short interpregnancy intervals, and failure to seek prenatal care. The role of behavioural factors is illuminated by the fact that, in developed countries, the risk of producing low-birth-weight infants declines sharply among mothers with 12 or more years of education.

The risk of giving birth to low-birth-weight infants is reduced among mothers who initiate prenatal care during the first three months of pregnancy. The main obstacles to prenatal care are similar in many different countries: a paucity of services in poor communities, attitudes that impede seeking help, inadequate transportation and child care, and lack of systems for caring for hard-to-reach women. In this important area of maternal and child health care, experience in technically advanced and developing countries can be exchanged to mutual advantage. To make substantial progress requires effective education for health; and this, in turn, requires collaboration between behavioural and biomedical sciences.

Diarrhoeal diseases remain one of the heaviest burdens of childhood illness throughout the developing world. Where studies of the use and impact of oral rehydration therapy have been made, the analysis has usually given inadequate attention to sociocultural factors. The ultimate health benefit of oral rehydration depends on its actual use, which, in turn, depends on the informed judgment of the mother. Her decision to use oral rehydration and her ability to use it effectively are influenced strongly by her social support system.

In any event, primary prevention is highly desirable. The main thrust of research indicates that the most effective interventions for diarrhoeal disease are those that interrupt the transmission of infectious agents in the home. There are well-documented findings concerning the importance of fecal contamination of food and water in the home. Controlled studies have shown the effectiveness of such simple actions as hand-washing in preventing infection. Changing behaviour for health in this domain can have powerful effects. However, the research literature on diarrhoeal diseases is weak in field studies on how to promote household hygiene in poor countries. Such studies, if adapted to different cultures and oriented toward health habits with long-term gains, could have substantial benefit in a relatively short time.

Studies in developing countries indicate that education has powerful effects on child health, nutrition, and fertility. Research has shown that the education of girls is a worthwhile investment in terms of a country's future economic growth and well-being, even where most women do not enter the labour force. Education delays marriage for women, partly by increasing their chances for employment; and educated women are more likely to know about and use contraceptives. Most girls in developing countries do, however, become mothers; and their influence on their children is crucial. At any particular income level, for example, the mother's educational level determines how well fed a family is. Moreover, studies in Asia, Africa, and Latin America have demonstrated that, even when differences in family income are taken into account, the more educated their mothers, the less likely are children to die.

Adolescence

The onset of adolescence is a critical period of biological and psychological change; puberty is one of the most far-reaching biological upheavals in the life span. For many, it involves drastic changes in the social environment as well. These years (10–15) are highly formative for health-relevant behaviour patterns such as smoking cigarettes, the use of alcohol or other drugs, driving automobiles and motorcycles, habits of food intake and exercise, and patterns of human relationships, including high-risk pregnancy and sexually transmitted disease. Before health-damaging patterns are firmly established, there is a crucial opportunity for preventive intervention.

Lessons can be learned from recent innovations and concomitant research in various parts of the world. For example, a number of studies have been carried out, in several countries, on preventing smoking, focusing mainly on 12- and 13-year-olds, a crucial time for the onset of smoking and other health-damaging behaviour. These studies show benefits of several years' duration. There is a clear decrease in smoking – of both cigarettes and marijuana – but also an unexpected tendency to reduce the use of alcohol and other drugs. The relevant programmes teach children how to resist peer pressure and other coping skills pertinent to major tasks of adolescent development.

Adolescence in humans – and in non-human primates – is a time when extensive changes occur in physiological and biochemical systems and behaviour. The basic mechanism of the neuroendocrine changes of puberty is of ancient origin and is essentially common to mammalian species. But, in humans, historically recent events have drastically altered the experience of adolescence, in some ways making it more difficult than ever before. Biological changes in humans over the past two centuries, induced by the control of infection and by better nutrition, particularly in affluent cultures, have lowered the average age of menarche. The trend for boys is similar, but harder to document. At the same time, the social changes occurring during these centuries have postponed the end of adolescence until much later. For many, this protracted period of adolescence introduces a high degree of uncertainty into their lives.

Although the human organism is reproductively mature in early adolescence, the brain does not reach a fully adult state of development until the end of the teenage years, and social maturity tends to lag behind mental maturity. Young adolescents, 10 to 15 years old, who are immature in knowledge, social experience, and cognitive development, make fateful decisions that can affect the entire course of their lives.

In premodern times, preparation for adulthood typically extended over much of childhood. Children had abundant opportunity to observe their parents and other adults performing the roles they themselves would eventually assume when the changes of puberty endowed them with an adult body and capabilities. The skills necessary for adult life were gradually acquired and fully available, or nearly so, by the end of puberty.

Today, there is probably more ambiguity and complexity about what constitutes preparation for effective adulthood than was ever the case before. Through most of human history, small societies have provided durable networks, familiar human relationships, and cultural guidance for young people, offering support in time of stress and teaching the skills necessary for coping and adaptation. In contemporary societies, such social support networks are being severely eroded because of extensive geographic mobility and migrations, the scattering of the extended family, and the rise of single-parent families, especially those involving very young, very poor, socially isolated mothers.

Adolescents are heavily exposed, particularly through the mass media, to sexuality, the use of alcohol and other drugs, smoking, reckless driving of vehicles, the use of weapons, and a variety of other temptations to engage in health-damaging behaviours. Although such 'diversions' may appear to young people to be casual, recreational, and tension-relieving, their effects endanger themselves and others.

Despite the drastic biological, social, and technical changes surrounding adolescence that have taken place since the Industrial Revolution, especially in this century, certain fundamental human needs appear to be enduring and crucial to survival and healthy development. These include the need to find a place in a valued group that provides a sense of belonging; the need to identify tasks that are generally recognized by the group as having adaptive value and that thus earn respect when skill in coping with them is acquired; the need to feel a sense of worth as a person; and the need for reliable and predictable relationships with other people, especially a few relatively close relationships.

The experience of industrialized nations suggests that rapid social changes, the breakdown of family supports, and the prolongation of adolescence are associated with an increase in behaviour-related problems such as substance abuse, school-age pregnancy, and educational failure. The opportunities for prevention rest heavily on finding constructive ways to meet the basic aspirations of adolescent development in a new social context.

It may be necessary to consider far-reaching changes in the preparation of young people for adult life, taking account of the drastic world transformation that has occurred and is still under way. Is it possible to provide teenagers with a basis for making wise decisions about the use of their own bodies and planning a constructive future? Is it possible to build social support networks in every community for stimulating interest, hope, and skills among young people and encouraging them to pursue education and protect their health?

Health and behaviour in developing countries: strengthening research capabilities

Some of the problems confronting nations today are the result of sociotechnical conditions that have appeared very recently in the evolution of the human species and that are changing at an accelerating rate. The magnitude and rate of these changes make it difficult to devise and implement solutions to human problems. This situation, formidable in the context of problems encountered within and among modern industrial societies, poses even larger obstacles to their solution in developing countries, in which the shift from old to new ways has been greatly compressed in time.

The rapid social changes of developing nations are having important effects on physical and mental health. These changes include massive urbanization, industrialization, large-scale migration, widespread unemployment and loss of self-esteem, prolongation of uncertainty about adult roles, a vast increase in the scale of the community of reference, and growing cultural heterogeneity and value conflict. Taken together, these factors tend to weaken traditional cultures and attenuate their socializing, orienting, and supportive functions. This, in turn, may have a significant impact on health-relevant behaviour, especially when the vital social functions are not assumed by other forces.

How can the technically advanced nations help to improve health in developing countries? One important priority is active collaboration in training competent personnel who can then develop and implement their own health-care systems. A second urgent need is support to the development of primary health-care networks, focusing particularly on maternal and child health. A third and crucial function is help in the conduct of research, research that is relevant to the needs of the developing countries, with special emphasis on ways in which patterns of living that protect against major risk factors can be introduced and fostered. Research in developing countries could usefully assess which principles and techniques of behavioural change promoting health in the developed world might be applicable to their own conditions, and how they can be adapted to specific cultures. If carefully designed, such investigations could serve as models for stimulating interest in community-based programmes and advance understanding of how such studies might be conducted in still other developing countries and applied to other problems.

It is important that mechanisms be developed for training indigenous health professionals and behavioural scientists in ways of carrying out specific, culturally sensitive studies on topics arising as problems in their work. From this emerges the great need to strengthen and expand the infrastructure that supports research in developing societies, including the institutional components essential to clinical and community research. It is equally important to establish exchange programs and collaborative relationships that not only allow local research workers to develop their skills but also keep them in touch with advances in health research in technically advanced societies. Collaborative research across national boundaries is especially important in this regard. There is ample evidence that collaboration in research can be beneficial for developing and technically advanced countries.

Can developing and developed countries alike, through research and community-based education, learn to adopt health-promoting behaviour and to avoid health-damaging behaviour? The experience of several countries gives reason for hope in this regard. Especially in the last decade, a major effort has been made to address the relationships of health and behaviour. In part, this has been done through informal education, and through the media. In significant part also, this effort has been carried forward by vigorous scientific inquiry. One promising approach has utilized information on risk factors in the population for cardiovascular and other diseases and the scientific study of behaviour, connecting this with biomedical research. The ability to change risk-factor behaviour toward health-promoting practices has been clearly demonstrated. In principle, such efforts can be applied to a variety of illnesses in the next decade; this will require sustained, cooperative efforts across disciplinary and national boundaries.

There is growing interest in cooperative efforts among nations to assess worldwide problems and to help developing countries adapt and apply technology to their own problems and circumstances. The success of such efforts will depend on the interaction between the use of technology and behaviour. The existence of technologies such as immunizations to deal with specific problems has typically not been sufficient to solve the problem. To be effective, methods for using and maintaining these technologies must be taught appropriately (taking cultural factors into account), understood adequately, and distributed widely. In health care, this requires linking epidemiology with the biomedical and behavioural sciences.

Mental health problems: the invisible pandemic
WHO has estimated that at least 300 million people in the world suffer from mental or neurological disorders or psychosocial problems such as alcohol and drug dependence (Sartorius, 1988). This estimate is probably too optimistic, since many epidemiological surveys done over the years indicate that the total prevalence of these disorders in a community is at least 8% to 10% of the population, which would give a total world estimate of 400–500 million people with such disorders. In developed countries, two of every five disabled persons are impaired because of these illnesses; and, as previously noted, as many as one in five contacts with health services worldwide can be traced back to a psychosocial problem.

What is clear today is that there is every likelihood that the number of these problems will increase in the years to come. This prediction rests on the rapid prolongation of life expectancy of those already disabled and the increasing proportion of the population at higher risk for mental and neurological disorders (e.g., schizophrenia with increased survival into young adulthood; depression in middle age; and dementia and stroke among the elderly because of a greater life expectancy of the general population).

The prediction of an increase in problems rests, however, on other supportive facts as well, at least two of which should be mentioned. The first is the continuing frustration of efforts to introduce broad-scale programmes that could prevent at least one-half of the problems now coming into existence. (WHO, 1988) The second is the continuing occurrence of diseases and problems that add to the number of those mentally ill. Earlier examples included damage to the central nervous system by new and powerful chemical substances and drugs and the increasing proportion of cases of malaria with significant cerebral involvement; the most recent examples are the neuropsychiatric syndromes linked to the acquired immunity deficiency syndrome (AIDS) and the AIDS-related complex.

At the same time, the last two decades have brought only modest advances in the treatment of mental and neurological disorders. Thus, in spite of the tremendous usefulness of the palliative treatments available today, mental and neurological disorders continue to cause misery and economic losses to the populations of the world.

The current rarity of highly qualified personnel in developing countries cannot be expected to change. Even if the total number of, say, psychiatrists in Africa were to double every year for the next ten years (which is unimaginable), there would still be five times fewer psychiatrists per population unit than we find today in the least-developed industrialized nations. Clearly, provision of adequate care must depend on other approaches. The two most likely to be useful are, first, acquiring more knowledge about mental and neurological disorders so as to be able to produce simple and effective methods of treatment and prevention of these disorders; and, second, involving the general health services in the care of the mentally ill. There is good evidence that this can be done efficiently.

Involving general health services, however, may not be enough: even if they are fully involved, much remains undone, as the experience of developed countries has demonstrated. The only way to deal with these other tasks is to bring in other social sectors and mobilize society at large in programmes aiming to help the mentally and neurologically ill. This mobilization is a major task, similar in nature to others that are facing public health authorities, who will have to become aware that public health cannot be improved if its psychosocial perspectives are neglected and the behaviour of individuals and human groups treated as a side issue rather than as a core element of all human progress.

It is the editors' hope that the papers assembled in this volume and the perspectives they offer on health and health-promotion programmes will stimulate researchers and make public health decision-makers aware of the central role of behaviour in the improvement of public health.

Notes

1. World Health Organization, Report of the second meeting of the Scientific Planning Group on the Expanded Programme of Research and Training in Biobehavioural Sciences and Mental Health (document ACMR24/82.12). World Health Organization, Geneva, 1982.
2. World Health Organization, Prevention of mental, neurological and psychosocial disorders. Report by the Director-General to the Thirty-ninth World Health Assembly (WHO document A39/9). World Health Organization, Geneva, 1986.

Bibliography

1. Hamburg, D. A., Elliott, G. R., & Parron, D. L. (Eds.). *Health and behaviour: Frontiers of research in the biobehavioural sciences.* Division of Mental Health and Behavioural Medicine, Institute of Medicine, National Academy of Sciences, Washington, DC, National Academy Press, 1982.
2. Lancaster, J. B. & Hamburg, B. A. (Eds.). *School-age Pregnancy and Parenthood: Biosocial Dimensions.* Social Sciences Research Council. Aldine de Gruyter, New York, 1986.
3. Institute of Medicine, National Academy of Sciences. *Preventing low birthweight.* Washington, DC. National Academy Press, 1985.
4. Institute of Medicine, National Academy of Sciences. *Confronting AIDS: Directions for public health, health care and research.* Washington, DC. National Academy Press, 1986.
5. Rohde, J. E. Acute diarrhoea, In: J. A. Walsh & K. S. Warren (Eds.). *Strategies for primary health care: Technologies appropriate for the control of disease in the developing world.* Chicago, University of Chicago Press, 1986.
6. Sartorius, N. 1987). Mental Health Policies and Programs for the Twenty-first Century: a Personal View. *Integrated Psychiatry,* **5**, 151–4.
7. Sartorius, N. The mental health programme of the World Health Organization, *Asia Pacific Journal of Public Health,* 1988, Vol. 2, No. 1.
8. UNICEF. *The state of the world's children, 1987.* New York, Oxford University Press, 1987.
9. UNICEF. *The state of the world's children, 1986.* New York, Oxford University Press, 1986.
10. US National Center for Health Statistics. *Health. United States, 1985* (DHHS Publications No. {PHS} 86-1232). Washington, DC, US Government Printing Office, 1985.

11. World Health Organization. (1981). Social Dimensions of Mental Health. WHO, Geneva.
12. World Health Organization. Biobehavioural and Mental Health Aspects of Primary Health Care with particular Emphasis on Maternal and Child Health: Research Possibilities: Report of a Task Force meeting, Washington, 29 August – 2 September 1983 (document MNH/83.29).
13. World Health Organization. Adaptation to Sociotechnical Change: Behavioural and Mental Health Implications: Report of a Task Force meeting, New Delhi, 15–21 December 1983 (document MNH/CHA/84.1).
14. World Health Organization. Alcohol-related Problems and their Prevention with particular Reference to Adolescence: Report of a Task Force meeting, Geneva, 31 August – 4 Sepetember 1984 (document MNH/NAT/84.1).

Index

221